Recent Titles in
Q&A Health Guides

Obesity: Your Questions Answered
Christine L. B. Selby

Birth Control: Your Questions Answered
Paul Quinn

Therapy and Counseling: Your Questions Answered
Christine L. B. Selby

Depression: Your Questions Answered
Romeo Vitelli

Food Labels: Your Questions Answered
Barbara A. Brehm

Smoking: Your Questions Answered
Stacy Mintzer Herlihy

Teen Stress: Your Questions Answered
Nicole Neda Zamanzadeh and Tamara D. Afifi

Grief and Loss: Your Questions Answered
Louis Kuykendall Jr.

Healthy Friendships: Your Questions Answered
Lauren Holleb

Trauma and Resilience: Your Questions Answered
Keith A. Young

Vegetarian and Vegan Diets: Your Questions Answered
Alice C. Richer

Yoga: Your Questions Answered
Anjali A. Sarkar

TEEN PREGNANCY

Your Questions Answered

Paul Quinn

Q&A Health Guides

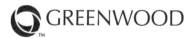

An Imprint of ABC-CLIO, LLC
Santa Barbara, California • Denver, Colorado

Library of Congress Cataloging-in-Publication Data

Names: Quinn, Paul, 1971– author.
Title: Teen pregnancy : your questions answered / Paul Quinn.
Description: Santa Barbara, California : Greenwood, [2021] | Series: Q&A
    health guides | Includes bibliographical references and index.
Identifiers: LCCN 2020036869 (print) | LCCN 2020036870 (ebook) |
    ISBN 9781440876110 (cloth) | ISBN 9781440876127 (ebook)
Subjects: LCSH: Teen pregnancy. | Childbirth—Miscellanea. |
    Pregnancy—Miscellanea.
Classification: LCC RG556.5 .Q85 2021 (print) | LCC RG556.5 (ebook) |
    DDC 618.200835—dc23
LC record available at https://lccn.loc.gov/2020036869
LC ebook record available at https://lccn.loc.gov/2020036870

ISBN: 978-1-4408-7611-0 (print)
       978-1-4408-7612-7 (ebook)

25 24 23 22 21   1 2 3 4 5

This book is also available as an eBook.

Greenwood
An Imprint of ABC-CLIO, LLC

ABC-CLIO, LLC
147 Castilian Drive
Santa Barbara, California 93117
www.abc-clio.com

This book is printed on acid-free paper ∞

Manufactured in the United States of America

To Mom and David—once more, and always

Contents

Series Foreword   xi

Acknowledgments   xiii

Introduction   xv

Guide to Health Literacy   xvii

Common Misconceptions about Teen Pregnancy   xxv

Questions and Answers   1

Teen Pregnancy as a Social Issue   3

   1. How common is teen pregnancy in the United States
     and around the world, and is teen pregnancy on the rise?   3
   2. What factors make someone more likely to become a
     teen parent?   4
   3. What societal factors influence teen pregnancy?   7
   4. What problems do teen parents face?   8
   5. What are the possible long-term effects for a child born
     to teen parents?   10
   6. What are the effects of teen pregnancy on a family?   11
   7. What are the consequences of teen pregnancy for
     society?   13

8. What impact have media portrayals had on perceptions
   of teen pregnancy and parenthood?   14
9. How can teen pregnancy be prevented?   17

Options for Pregnant Teens   21

10. What do I do if I decide to have an abortion?   21
11. Are there different types of abortions, and how far into a
    pregnancy is each type available?   23
12. What are the costs associated with an abortion?   27
13. What are the possible complications of an abortion?   30
14. Can I get an abortion without telling my parents?   32
15. How does the adoption process work?   33
16. Are there different types of adoption?   35
17. If I decide to keep my baby, what do I need to provide
    my child with once it's born?   37
18. What resources are available if I decide to keep
    the baby?   38
19. What financial assistance is available to teen mothers
    and their children?   40
20. What do I do if I keep the baby and then I can't handle
    things anymore?   41

Pregnancy, Delivery, and Medical Concerns for Teens   43

21. How do the menstrual cycle and conception work?   43
22. How can I tell if I'm pregnant?   44
23. Is teen pregnancy dangerous?   46
24. What can I expect to happen in each trimester?   48
25. Will I need any special prenatal care?   50
26. Are my baby and I covered under my parents' health
    insurance?   52
27. How will I know if I'm in labor?   53
28. What can I expect when it's time to deliver the baby?   56
29. Can I have a normal birth, or do I have to have a
    cesarean birth?   59
30. Am I at risk for any complications because I'm a
    teenager?   61
31. Is my baby at risk for any medical complications
    because I'm a teenager?   63
32. What medical care does the baby need after it's born?   64
33. Will I be able to breastfeed?   66
34. How do I prevent getting pregnant again?   68

35. Does having a baby in my teens affect my ability to have
    children in the future?   70
36. Are there any mental or emotional concerns I need
    to worry about during pregnancy or after giving birth?   72

Legal Concerns   75

37. Do I have to tell my parents I'm pregnant?   75
38. Do my parents have to be involved in any decisions
    I make regarding the pregnancy?   76
39. Are my parents legally required to take care of me and
    my baby?   78
40. Do I have to get married because I'm pregnant or got
    someone pregnant?   80
41. What rights and responsibilities does the baby's
    father have?   81
42. Can the baby's father get custody of the baby?   83
43. What are the legal implications of a pregnancy caused
    by rape or incest?   85
44. What can happen if the mother is a minor and the
    father of the baby is a legal adult?   89
45. Can my baby be taken away from me because
    I'm a teenager?   90

Other Concerns   93

46. What do I do if I don't know who the father is?   93
47. How does a paternity test work?   94
48. Will people be able to tell that I'm pregnant?   96
49. Will my pregnancy affect my current or future
    relationships?   98
50. Will my social life change because I'm pregnant?   100
51. What do I do if my parents kick me out of the house?   101
52. Can I quit school and get a job?   103
53. Will I be able to finish school if I have a baby?   105
54. Will I be able to go to college if I have a baby
    in my teens?   108

Case Studies   111

Glossary   125

Directory of Resources   135

Index   141

Series Foreword

All of us have questions about our health. Is this normal? Should I be doing something differently? Whom should I talk to about my concerns? And our modern world is full of answers. Thanks to the Internet, there's a wealth of information at our fingertips, from forums where people can share their personal experiences to Wikipedia articles to the full text of medical studies. But finding the right information can be an intimidating and difficult task—some sources are written at too high a level, others have been oversimplified, while still others are heavily biased or simply inaccurate.

Q&A Health Guides address the needs of readers who want accurate, concise answers to their health questions, authored by reputable and objective experts, and written in clear and easy-to-understand language. This series focuses on the topics that matter most to young adult readers, including various aspects of physical and emotional well-being as well as other components of a healthy lifestyle. These guides will also serve as a valuable tool for parents, school counselors, and others who may need to answer teens' health questions.

All books in the series follow the same format to make finding information quick and easy. Each volume begins with an essay on health literacy and why it is so important when it comes to gathering and evaluating health information. Next, the top five myths and misconceptions that surround the topic are dispelled. The heart of each guide is a collection of questions and answers, organized thematically. A selection of five case studies provides real-world examples to illuminate key concepts. Rounding out each volume are a directory of resources, glossary, and index.

It is our hope that the books in this series will not only provide valuable information but will also help guide readers toward a lifetime of healthy decision making.

Acknowledgments

This work would not be possible without the support and encouragement from my family, friends, and colleagues. Specifically, sincere thanks and appreciation to Eileen Guidice, David Gilsenan, "Maggie and Milo," Tina Neri-Badame, Gregory Locoparra, Denise & Ty Mojica, Mary Quinn, Kelly & Tom Greco, Joe & Gail Guidice, Anthony & Laura Guidice, Roxanne Guidice, Donna Petrolia, John & Mindy Gilsenan, Mike & Mary Lanni, Christine Lanni, Michael & Alyssa Lanni, John & Gina Nicoletti-Gilsenan, Kate & Marwan Amaisse, Matt Gilsenan, and the memory of Gladys Gilsenan and Maryanne Hedrick. In addition, Robert Velez, Larry Lane, Joel Kunkel, Jim McCoy, Jeffrey Cervone-Bonamo, Sean & Marie Sherrock, Ian Klein, Felipe Guzman, Marvin Kasper, Ann Marie Leichman, Charles Vannoy, Peter Jarosz and my friends, and coworkers and colleagues of The Valley Health System were a constant source of support and encouragement.

Social workers and care managers are the unsung heroes of health care. I remain extremely grateful for the expertise and guidance of Terry Grueter, Erin Smith, Nina Halstead, and Nadine Morton.

Unexpected turns happen in life. I am sincerely grateful for the expertise, skill, and compassion of Dr. Michael Passeri, Dr. Kevin Wood, and Dr. Anna Korcis for taking care of who matters most to me.

I remain extremely grateful to Maxine Taylor, Lettie Conrad, and Tracey Molineaux for their literary, publishing, and promotional expertise and direction.

Some people never get to meet their heroes or guardian angel—I was raised with mine. Thank you, Vinny, for the spirit that pushes me to do more and be more than I ever imagined.

Finally, I can do this work only because of the invaluable lessons I have learned from the men and women I have had the honor to care for, my patients, during close to three decades of nursing and midwifery practice. Your lives, stories, resilience, and spirit are forever part of my soul.

Introduction

It is estimated that 3 in 10 girls will become pregnant at least once before age 20. With 750,000 teen pregnancies occurring each year, 18.8% of teen girls age 15 to 19, then, are likely to be pregnant. The issue of teen pregnancy, however, is a global phenomenon. Although rates of teen pregnancy are beginning to decline, rates of teen pregnancy remain high in specific racial groups like Hispanics (28.9%), and non-Hispanic blacks (27.5%) compared to non-Hispanic white teen girls (13.2%). Thus, the World Health Organization estimates that about 16 million girls between the ages of 15 to 19, and about 1 million girls younger than age 15, give birth each year. As the global population of adolescent girls continue to grow, so do the chances that more teen girls (and teen boys as fathers) will become pregnant by 2030.

Teens are having their first sexual encounters, including sexual intercourse, as early as junior high or grammar school in the United States. There is a belief, perhaps popularized by social media, television, or the movies that dating, relationships, and intimacy signify maturity, worthiness, acceptance, or popularity. Teens who have sex at younger ages often lack access to a proper and consistent form of birth control and are highly susceptible to pregnancy. There is no single risk factor that makes a teen more likely to become a parent. Multiple factors influence teen pregnancy. Teens are beginning, and engaging in, sexual activity regularly and at young ages. Contraceptive access and options are limited for most teens.

Families, further, have a significant impact on a teen's self-esteem and set the example for mature relationships between adults. An environment of poverty, few resources, violence, drug or alcohol abuse, peer pressure, and teens being surrounded by teens who are all sexually active can also increase the likelihood of teens becoming parents.

Teen pregnancy is a significant issue for society. Teen parents require significant resources and support. Babies and children of teen parents also require financial, social, and educational resources to allow then to develop into mature adults who contribute to society. Without help, teen parents often perpetuate the cycle of poverty and will likely raise a child who will become a teen parent themselves. Significant health risks accompany teen pregnancy, for both mother and baby, that can also challenge a family's, or a society's, resources.

There is no single strategy or tactic that will mitigate, or fix, the global dilemma posed by teen pregnancy. However, teens have demonstrated their abilities to be successful parents and become productive members of society. The objective of this book is to break down the stigma surrounding teen pregnancy and provide a comprehensive exploration of the issues, influences, and suggestions for individuals, families, communities, or societies. By providing information and education in a simple format regarding teen pregnancy, this book answers important common questions people have regarding teen pregnancy. Furthermore, this book can be used to stimulate honest, open communication between teens, parents, health care practitioners, and others to provide guidance about health care, legal, or social issues surrounding teen pregnancy. Sex, and sexual activity, carry no shame; however, irresponsible unprotected sex or sexual activity, or abusive, illegal, or antiquated traditions or cultural norms can have deleterious outcomes for a growing population of young people, their babies or children, and society. This book explores a topic many people are too ashamed, afraid, embarrassed, or uncomfortable to ask, using the most recent, accurate scientific evidence available in easy-to-understand language.

---------------◆:◆---------------

Guide to Health Literacy

On her 13th birthday, Samantha was diagnosed with type 2 diabetes. She consulted her mom and her aunt, both of whom also have type 2 diabetes, and decided to go with their strategy of managing diabetes by taking insulin. As a result of participating in an after-school program at her middle school that focused on health literacy, she learned that she can help manage the level of glucose in her bloodstream by counting her carbohydrate intake, following a diabetic diet, and exercising regularly. But, what exactly should she do? How does she keep track of her carbohydrate intake? What is a diabetic diet? How long should she exercise and what type of exercise should she do? Samantha is a visual learner, so she turned to her favorite source of media, YouTube, to answer these questions. She found videos from individuals around the world sharing their experiences and tips, doctors (or at least people who have "Dr." in their YouTube channel names), government agencies such as the National Institutes of Health, and even video clips from cat lovers who have cats with diabetes. With guidance from the librarian and the health and science teachers at her school, she assessed the credibility of the information in these videos and even compared their suggestions to some of the print resources that she was able to find at her school library. Now, she knows exactly how to count her carbohydrate level, how to prepare and follow a diabetic diet, and how much (and what) exercise is needed daily. She intends to share her findings with her mom and her aunt, and now she wants to create a chart that summarizes what she has learned that she can share with her doctor.

Samantha's experience is not unique. She represents a shift in our society; an individual no longer views himself or herself as a passive recipient of medical care but as an active mediator of his or her own health. However, in this era when any individual can post his or her opinions and experiences with a particular health condition online with just a few clicks or publish a memoir, it is vital that people know how to assess the credibility of health information. Gone are the days when "publishing" health information required intense vetting. The health information landscape is highly saturated, and people have innumerable sources where they can find information about practically any health topic. The sources (whether print, online, or a person) that an individual consults for health information are crucial because the accuracy and trustworthiness of the information can potentially affect his or her overall health. The ability to find, select, assess, and use health information constitutes a type of literacy—health literacy—that everyone must possess.

THE DEFINITION AND PHASES OF HEALTH LITERACY

One of the most popular definitions for health literacy comes from Ratzan and Parker (2000), who describe health literacy as "the degree to which individuals have the capacity to obtain, process, and understand basic health information and services needed to make appropriate health decisions." Recent research has extrapolated health literacy into health literacy bits, further shedding light on the multiple phases and literacy practices that are embedded within the multifaceted concept of health literacy. Although this research has focused primarily on online health information seeking, these health literacy bits are needed to successfully navigate both print and online sources. There are six phases of health information seeking: (1) Information Need Identification and Question Formulation, (2) Information Search, (3) Information Comprehension, (4) Information Assessment, (5) Information Management, and (6) Information Use.

The first phase is the *information need identification and question formulation phase*. In this phase, one needs to be able to develop and refine a range of questions to frame one's search and understand relevant health terms. In the second phase, *information search*, one has to possess appropriate searching skills, such as using proper keywords and correct spelling in search terms, especially when using search engines and databases. It is also crucial to understand how search engines work (i.e., how search results are derived, what the order of the search results means, how to use the snippets that are provided in the search results list to select websites, and how to determine which listings are ads on a search engine results page). One also has to limit reliance on surface characteristics, such as the design of a website or a book (a website or book that appears to have a lot of information or looks aesthetically pleasant does not necessarily mean it has good information) and language used (a website or book that utilizes jargon, the keywords that one used to conduct the search, or the word "information" does not necessarily indicate it will have good information). The next phase is *information comprehension*, whereby one needs to have the ability to read, comprehend, and recall the information (including textual, numerical, and visual content) one has located from the books and/or online resources.

To assess the credibility of health information (*information assessment* phase), one needs to be able to evaluate information for accuracy, evaluate how current the information is (e.g., when a website was last updated or when a book was published), and evaluate the creators of the source—for example, examine site sponsors or type of sites (.com, .gov, .edu, or .org) or the author of a book (practicing doctor, a celebrity doctor, a patient of a specific disease, etc.) to determine the believability of the person/organization providing the information. Such credibility perceptions tend to become generalized, so they must be frequently reexamined (e.g., the belief that a specific news agency always has credible health information needs continuous vetting). One also needs to evaluate the credibility of the medium (e.g., television, Internet, radio, social media, and book) and evaluate—not just accept without questioning—others' claims regarding the validity of a site, book, or other specific source of information. At this stage, one has to "make sense of information gathered from diverse sources by identifying misconceptions, main and supporting ideas, conflicting information, point of view, and biases" (American Association of School Librarians [AASL], 2009, p. 13) and conclude which sources/information are valid and accurate by using conscious strategies rather than simply using intuitive judgments or "rules of thumb." This phase is the most challenging segment of health information seeking and serves as a determinant of success (or lack thereof) in the information-seeking process. The following section on Sources of Health Information further explains this phase.

The fifth phase is *information management*, whereby one has to organize information that has been gathered in some manner to ensure easy retrieval and use in the future. The last phase is *information use*, in which one will synthesize information found across various resources, draw conclusions, and locate the answer to his or her original question and/or the content that fulfills the information need. This phase also often involves implementation, such as using the information to solve a health problem; make health-related decisions; identify and engage in behaviors that will help a person to avoid health risks; share the health information found with family members and friends who may benefit from it; and advocate more broadly for personal, family, or community health.

THE IMPORTANCE OF HEALTH LITERACY

The conception of health has moved from a passive view (someone is either well or ill) to one that is more active and process based (someone is working toward preventing or managing disease). Hence, the dominant focus has shifted from doctors and treatments to patients and prevention, resulting in the need to strengthen our ability and confidence (as patients and consumers of health care) to look for, assess, understand, manage, share, adapt, and use health-related information. An individual's health literacy level has been found to predict his or her health status better than age, race, educational attainment, employment status, and income level (National Network of Libraries of Medicine, 2013). Greater health literacy also enables individuals to better communicate with health care providers such as doctors, nutritionists, and therapists, as they can pose more relevant, informed, and useful questions to health care providers. Another added advantage of greater health literacy is better information-seeking skills, not only for health but also in other domains, such as completing assignments for school.

SOURCES OF HEALTH INFORMATION:
THE GOOD, THE BAD, AND THE IN-BETWEEN

For generations, doctors, nurses, nutritionists, health coaches, and other health professionals have been the trusted sources of health information. Additionally, researchers have found that young adults, when they have health-related questions, typically turn to a family member who has had firsthand experience with a health condition because of their family member's close proximity and because of their past experience with, and trust in, this individual. Expertise should be a core consideration when consulting a person, website, or book for health information. The credentials and background of the person or author and conflicting interests of the author (and his or her organization) must be checked and validated to ensure the likely credibility of the health information they are conveying. While books often have implied credibility because of the peer-review process involved, self-publishing has challenged this credibility, so qualifications of book authors should also be verified. When it comes to health information, currency of the source must also be examined. When examining health information/studies presented, pay attention to the exhaustiveness of research methods utilized to offer recommendations or conclusions. Small and nondiverse sample size is often—but not always—an indication of reduced credibility. Studies that confuse correlation with causation is another potential issue to watch for. Information seekers must also pay attention to the sponsors of the research studies. For example, if a study is sponsored by manufacturers of drug Y and the study recommends that drug Y is the best treatment to manage or cure a disease, this may indicate a lack of objectivity on the part of the researchers.

The Internet is rapidly becoming one of the main sources of health information. Online forums, news agencies, personal blogs, social media sites, pharmacy sites, and celebrity "doctors" are all offering medical and health information targeted to various types of people in regard to all types of diseases and symptoms. There are professional journalists, citizen journalists, hoaxers, and people paid to write fake health news on various sites that may appear to have a legitimate domain name and may even have authors who claim to have professional credentials, such as an MD. All these sites *may* offer useful information or information that appears to be useful and relevant; however, much of the information may be debatable and may fall into gray areas that require readers to discern credibility, reliability, and biases.

While broad recognition and acceptance of certain media, institutions, and people often serve as the most popular determining factors to assess credibility of health information among young people, keep in mind that there are legitimate Internet sites, databases, and books that publish health information and serve as sources of health information for doctors, other health sites, and members of the public. For example, MedlinePlus (https://medlineplus.gov) has trusted sources on over 975 diseases and conditions and presents the information in easy-to-understand language.

The chart here presents factors to consider when assessing credibility of health information. However, keep in mind that these factors function only as a guide and require continuous updating to keep abreast with the changes in the landscape of health information, information sources, and technologies.

The chart can serve as a guide; however, approaching a librarian about how one can go about assessing the credibility of both print and online health information is far more effective than using generic checklist-type tools. While librarians are not health experts, they can apply and teach patrons strategies to determine the credibility of health information.

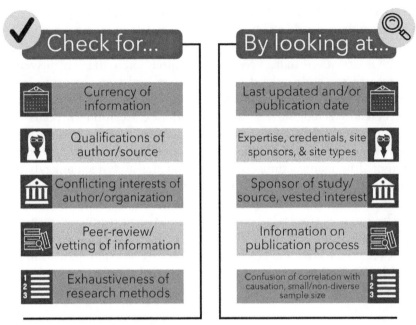

All images from flaticon.com

With the prevalence of fake sites and fake resources that appear to be legitimate, it is important to use the following health information assessment tips to verify health information that one has obtained (St. Jean et al., 2015, p. 151):

- **Don't assume you are right**: Even when you feel very sure about an answer, keep in mind that the answer may not be correct, and it is important to conduct (further) searches to validate the information.
- **Don't assume you are wrong**: You may actually have correct information, even if the information you encounter does not match—that is, you may be right and the resources that you have found may contain false information.
- **Take an open approach**: Maintain a critical stance by not including your preexisting beliefs as keywords (or letting them influence your choice of keywords) in a search, as this may influence what it is possible to find out.
- **Verify, verify, and verify**: Information found, especially on the Internet, needs to be validated, no matter how the information appears on the site (i.e., regardless of the appearance of the site or the quantity of information that is included).

Health literacy comes with experience navigating health information. Professional sources of health information, such as doctors, health care providers, and health databases, are still the best, but one also has the power to search for health information and then verify it by consulting with these trusted sources and by using the health information assessment tips and guide shared previously.

Mega Subramaniam, PhD
Associate Professor, College of Information Studies,
University of Maryland

REFERENCES AND FURTHER READING

American Association of School Librarians (AASL). (2009). *Standards for the 21st-century learner in action.* Chicago, IL: American Association of School Librarians.

Hilligoss, B., & Rieh, S.-Y. (2008). Developing a unifying framework of credibility assessment: Construct, heuristics, and interaction in context. *Information Processing & Management, 44*(4), 1467–1484.

Kuhlthau, C. C. (1988). Developing a model of the library search process: Cognitive and affective aspects. *Reference Quarterly, 28*(2), 232–242.

National Network of Libraries of Medicine (NNLM). (2013). Health literacy. Bethesda, MD: National Network of Libraries of Medicine. Retrieved from nnlm.gov/outreach/consumer/hlthlit.html

Ratzan, S. C., & Parker, R. M. (2000). Introduction. In C. R. Selden, M. Zorn, S. C. Ratzan, & R. M. Parker (Eds.), *National Library of Medicine current bibliographies in medicine: Health literacy.* NLM Pub. No. CBM 2000-1. Bethesda, MD: National Institutes of Health, U.S. Department of Health and Human Services.

St. Jean, B., Taylor, N. G., Kodama, C., & Subramaniam, M. (February 2017). Assessing the health information source perceptions of tweens using card-sorting exercises. *Journal of Information Science.* Retrieved from http://journals.sagepub.com/doi/abs/10.1177/01655515 16687728

St. Jean, B., Subramaniam, M., Taylor, N. G., Follman, R., Kodama, C., & Casciotti, D. (2015). The influence of positive hypothesis testing on youths' online health-related information seeking. *New Library World, 116*(3/4), 136–154.

Subramaniam, M., St. Jean, B., Taylor, N. G., Kodama, C., Follman, R., & Casciotti, D. (2015). Bit by bit: Using design-based research to improve the health literacy of adolescents. *JMIR Research Protocols,*

4(2), paper e62. Retrieved from http://www.ncbi.nlm.nih.gov/pmc
/articles/PMC4464334/
Valenza, J. (2016, November 26). Truth, truthiness, and triangulation: A
news literacy toolkit for a "post-truth" world [Web log]. Retrieved from
http://blogs.slj.com/neverendingsearch/2016/11/26/truth-truthiness
-triangulation-and-the-librarian-way-a-news-literacy-toolkit-for-a
-post-truth-world/

Common Misconceptions about Teen Pregnancy

1. ONLY GIRLS FROM LOWER SOCIOECONOMIC CLASSES GET PREGNANT AS TEENS

Globally, teen pregnancy is a problem that occurs in high-, middle-, and low-income countries. Teen pregnancies are more likely to occur in marginalized communities, commonly driven by poverty, lack of education, and employment opportunities. Although many personal, social, and family factors influence a teen becoming a parent, factors in the teen's physical environment, living conditions, the community, and its resources all contribute toward influencing if a teen becomes a parent. Communities who fail to provide adequate schooling, or communities where teens stop attending or do not complete school, are more likely to have more teens who are unemployed or underemployed in jobs with low income. Lack of adequate financial resources (e.g., coming from a low-income family, living in poverty, or being homeless) are also contributing factors toward teen pregnancy. Teens who live in neighborhoods with neighborhood unrest like violence, gang activity, visible evidence of drug use, or run-down buildings often live in fear, can be easily intimidated by, or suffer abuses from, peers or other people in the community. The combined lack of resources, employment, and housing contributes to teens being more likely to engage in, or be forced into, unprotected sexual activity that could lead to parenthood. Being in the welfare or foster care system can also impact teen pregnancy. Teens who move from foster home to foster home, or who are locked into the welfare system as their only means of any financial support or other resources are more likely to become teen parents. For more information, see Questions 1–3 and 49–54.

2. TEEN BOYS HAVE NO RESPONSIBILITY IF THEIR GIRLFRIEND BECOMES PREGNANT

Teen fathers have rights and responsibilities as a parent. While the teen mother is pregnant and the baby is unborn, however, a teen father has no rights to control any decision a teen mother makes about her own health, including if she opts to have an abortion. After the baby is born, a teen father has the right to sue for, and confirm via, a paternity test that he is indeed the father of the baby and, if he is the father, to have access to his baby through regular visitation or a custody arrangement and be involved in the baby's life. A teen father is responsible to pay child support and to maintain a lifestyle or employment that permits him to make those payments. A teen father has the responsibility to spend time with his child, be interested in and participate in their child's life, to keep them from harm, and provide them a safe environment to grow and flourish. As a role model for the child, a teen father has the responsibility to finish their education or obtain a graduate equivalency diploma (GED), get vocational training or attend college, and make wise choices about who they permit in their social circle or the interests or activities they participate in. Aside from the information covered in Question 41, see also Questions 42–44 for additional information.

3. ABORTION IS THE ONLY RECOURSE A TEENAGE GIRL HAS IF SHE BECOMES PREGNANT

A teenage girl has three options to consider if she becomes pregnant: she can have an abortion and end the pregnancy, complete the pregnancy and raise her child, or complete the pregnancy and put the baby up for adoption. Although abortions are common, they can only be performed during a limited time early in the pregnancy and have significant risks for physical and emotional complications or consequences. If a mother opts to keep her baby, she will need multiple resources, including support from her family or the father of the baby, to provide for her child's various needs. There are different types of adoption processes available to a teen mother depending on the type of access, involvement, or anonymity she wishes to have in her child's life. For additional information, see Questions 10–20, 38, and 41.

4. TEENAGERS CANNOT BE GOOD PARENTS

Teenagers can be great parents! Although the vast majority of research demonstrates that children born to teen parents face numerous challenges and obstacles, teen parents love their children unconditionally and strive to do what is best for their child just like adult parents. Teens try to keep a positive attitude and want to spend quality time with their child. Teens are also more likely to be accepting of their situation and, if the pregnancy was viewed or considered a mistake, they work to make things better for the future. Teen parents are also receptive to learning or education and can be taught essential skills to make them good parents. Teens know how to make a child feel valued and can teach children the difference between right and wrong. Teens can also create a nurturing environment for a child so he or she can thrive and grow into a confident, independent adult in the future. Having a child at a young age does not stop either of the young parents from fulfilling their dreams or attaining success in life. However, these things become more difficult because of the extra responsibility of taking care of the baby. However, a teen's resources are limited and, despite their best intentions, can face many difficulties raising their child. A teen's chances of becoming a successful parent increases if they had good parents who role modeled proper parenting behaviors. Therefore, adequate family, social, and financial support allows them to be good parents. For more information see Questions 4–8 and 17–19.

5. TEEN PARENTS CAN NEVER FINISH HIGH SCHOOL OR GO TO COLLEGE

Pregnant teens often perceive that caring for their baby or child is more important than obtaining or completing their education. Researchers conclude that most pregnant teens drop out of high school because of the fear of embarrassment, humiliation, and harassment from the fellow friends or peers. However, federal and state programs exist to help teens finish high school. Title IX requires schools to excuse absences for pregnancy, childbirth, or related conditions. It provides teen mothers the opportunity to stay in school and complete their education. It requires schools to provide pregnant students with the same services and accommodations equal to those provided to nonpregnant students (e.g., homeschooling, tutoring, independent study) or attend a separate program for pregnant and parenting students if they wish. Other schools offer innovative programs to help teens complete high school like on- site day care, home-school options, tutoring, or virtual courses. In some states Temporary Assistance for Needy Families (TANF) programs may provide additional benefits like child care assistance, help with obtaining a graduate equivalency diploma (GED) or vocational training. Pregnant teens can also go on to complete college education. Teens may postpone going to college to care for the baby or to save money for tuition. Colleges now offer more variety in their course offerings like online programs, night school, or weekend programs that allow teen parents to work at their own pace to complete college education. Often financial assistance programs are available. For more information see Questions 7, 9, 18, 53, and 54.

QUESTIONS AND ANSWERS

Teen Pregnancy as a Social Issue

1. How common is teen pregnancy in the United States and around the world, and is teen pregnancy on the rise?

It is estimated that 3 in 10 teen girls will become pregnant at least once before age 20. That means that 750,000 teen pregnancies occur each year. According to the Centers for Disease Control and Prevention (CDC), a total of 194,377 babies were born to women aged 15 to 19 in 2017, producing a birthrate of 18.8% per 1,000 women in this age group. Although there is a noticeable drop in the rate of teen girls becoming pregnant in the United States, the global teen pregnancy rate remains substantially high. The issues are also not limited to teen girls who become pregnant; teenage boys are becoming fathers, naturally, at the same rate as girls.

In the United States, teen pregnancy rates remain high among specific racial groups. For example, birthrates for Hispanic teens (i.e., 28.9%) and non-Hispanic black teens (27.5%) were more than two times higher than the rate for non-Hispanic white teens (13.2%). Geographic differences in teen birthrates persist, both within and across the United States. According to data from 2017, the state with the highest teen birthrate was Arkansas; for every 1,000 females between the ages of 15 and 19, 32.8% gave birth. Mississippi came in second place with 31 teen births per every 1,000 females. Oklahoma rounded out the top three with 29.7% teen births per every 1,000 women per year. In contrast,

Connecticut, New Hampshire, and Massachusetts had the lowest teen pregnancy rates.

Globally, teen pregnancy is a problem that occurs in high-, middle-, and low-income countries. Teen pregnancies are more likely to occur in marginalized communities, commonly driven by poverty, lack of education, and employment opportunities. For some, pregnancy and childbirth are planned and wanted. In addition, some countries force girls to marry and have children, while in other countries pregnancy is neither wanted nor planned due to lack of access to contraception.

Teen pregnancy is highest in the countries in Africa. For example, the country of Niger reports 203 births per every 1,000 teen women, followed by Mali (175 per 1,000 teen women), Angola (166 per 1,000 teen women), Mozambique (142 per 1,000 teen women), Guinea (141 per 1,000 teen women), Chad (131 per 1,000 teen women), and Malawi (136 per 1,000 teen women). In several of these countries, teenage marriages are the leading cause of subsequent teen pregnancies.

Thus, teen pregnancy remains a worldwide phenomenon. It is estimated that 11% of all births globally occur to women 15 to 19 years old. According to the World Health Organization (WHO), about 16 million girls between the ages of 15 to 19, and about 1 million girls younger than 15, give birth each year. Therefore, an estimated 21 million girls aged 15 to 19 and 2 million under the age of 15 become pregnant in developing regions. Despite a general decrease in births to teen mothers between the years 1990–2015, the global population of adolescents, especially girls, continues to grow. Projections by the WHO indicate that the number of adolescent pregnancies will increase globally for both boys and girls as teen parents by the year 2030, with the greatest increases in West, Central, Eastern and Southern Africa, Latin America, and the industrialized Western and European nations. Thus, teens as parents are becoming a true international concern.

2. What factors make someone more likely to become a teen parent?

Teen pregnancy can occur in any family or culture. Although the incidence of teen pregnancy in the United States is showing promising signs of decline, it still occurs, and remains a global health concern. There is no single risk factor that would make a teen more likely to become a parent; indeed, there are individual, family, and social factors that can contribute to someone becoming a teen parent for both boys and girls.

Individual Factors

There are multiple factors that could predispose a teen to becoming a parent. One of the primary factors is drug and alcohol use. Drugs and alcohol, when used alone or in combination, alter a person's sensations, decision making, and judgment. Teens using drugs and/or alcohol are more likely to participate in impulsive behavior and less likely to use contraception with each sexual encounter. Despite the multiple contraceptive options available, teens lack knowledge about each option or about which option would work best for them. In addition, many methods, for example, oral contraceptive or birth control pills, require a physical examination and a prescription from a health care practitioner; a teen may not have easy access to those services nor the funds to purchase contraception. Teens may also be reluctant or embarrassed to seek help with contraception options. There may also be a negative attitude toward using contraception. Teens who do not believe in using contraception for religious, moral, or social reasons, or those who do not believe that contraception is effective, are less likely to use it; thus, the likelihood of pregnancy occurring with episodes of unprotected sexual activity increases.

Teens who struggle with self-esteem issues may seek validation or define themselves as good, worthy, smart, or strong through their intimate relationships, including engaging in sexual activity. Further, teens who perform poorly in school may use sexual activity to feel successful, smart, or empowered. In contrast, some teens may feel ambivalent about having a child. Teens who either believe becoming a parent cannot happen to them, or that a pregnancy would not be an issue if it occurs, are more likely to participate in impulsive, unprotected sexual activity.

Having sexual activity at a young age also increases the likelihood of teen pregnancy. The earlier a teen initiates and sustains sexual activity, the higher the likelihood of the teen becoming a parent. Thus, teen pregnancy is likely with repeated episodes of unprotected sex. Having sex at a young age may not always be consensual. Teens who suffer with sexual abuse, or those who experience both incest and nonfamilial abuse, are more likely to become teen parents. Sexual abuse can alter perceptions about sexual behavior and influences the teen's judgment in forming intimate relationships, leading to earlier sexual debut, more sexual partners, and increased risk of sexual violence.

Family Factors

The family system that surrounds a teen can directly impact a teen's likelihood of becoming a teen parent. Parents who do not monitor their teen's whereabouts, social circle, school performance, social media activity, or behavior are more likely to have a teen who may engage in impulsive, unprotected sexual activity. When teens feel embarrassed, afraid, or otherwise reluctant to discuss any fears, concerns, or questions about sexual activity, and where poor communication exists between the teen and the parents, are more likely to have a teen who may become a parent. Open, honest, supportive dialogue between parents and teens promotes trust and support for issues or questions surrounding sexual activity with a partner.

Teens who fight with, are intimidated by, or fearful of parents or other family members and have negative family interactions may seek support, comfort, or validation through sexual activity with a partner. Teens in a single-parent family may lack the supervision of the parent, or have negative interactions with the parent, thus leading to an increased likelihood of the teen engaging in early, or frequent, sexual activity. Teens who are raised in families where a teen pregnancy has occurred, where a teen has become a parent, or where teens becoming parents is common or viewed as normal, are more likely to become parents themselves.

Social Factors

A teen's social circle, or the environment a teen lives in, can impact the likelihood of a teen becoming a parent. Teens are easily susceptible to the opinions or suggestions of their peers, including whether sexual activity is acceptable or encouraged. Teens whose friends are engaging in sexual activity are more likely to be sexually active themselves. Teens who feel isolated from their peer group, have poor peer relationships, have few friends, or experience bullying or threatening behavior from peers or classmates are more likely to seek support, acceptance, or validation from their intimate relationships. Sexual activity could be a way to preserve an intimate relationship or to experience feelings of love, acceptance, or approval.

Teens begin expanding their friendship networks and meet new people. As teens 13 to 15 years old begin to date and have new romantic relationships, the likelihood of them engaging in sexual activity without the use of contraception increases. Teens who date people older than themselves may feel a sense of maturity or a need to act more like their older partner, including the need to engage in sexual activity.

3. What societal factors influence teen pregnancy?

The environment that a teen lives in has a direct impact on their like-lihood of becoming a teen parent. Although many personal, social, and family factors influence a teen becoming a parent, factors in the teen's physical environment, living conditions, the community, and its resources all contribute toward influencing if a teen becomes a parent.

High unemployment within the community has been identified to impact teen pregnancy. Work, and adhering to a regular work schedule, not only provides financial benefits like money to purchase basic needs but also pro-motes benefits like personal growth, satisfaction, self-esteem, and social inter-actions. When people, including teens, are not working or attending school, there is increased unproductive time to engage in other activities, including sex, to relieve boredom, provide distraction, or to achieve a sense of worth. Further, people who work and develop a career are more likely to postpone parenthood until their personal, educational, or financial goals are met.

Poor or inadequate education for teens can also impact teen pregnancy. Education is empowering. Communities who fail to provide adequate schooling, or communities where teens stop attending or do not complete school, are more likely to have more teens that are unemployed or under-employed in jobs with low income. Further, a teen who lives in a home where parents or older siblings have not completed their education or who do not support the teen to advance their education is more likely to have a poor, or incomplete, education.

Lack of adequate financial resources (e.g., coming from a low-income family, living in poverty, or being homeless) are also contributing factors toward teen pregnancy. Families without financial resources or a means to sustain day-to-day living struggle. Teens in these environments are more likely to turn to unprotected sexual activity.

Neighborhoods where teens have no safe place to go for socialization or where there are few neighborhood opportunities for youth involvement are more likely to find alternative, often unsuitable, places to hang out or groups to associate with. Within these groups, the potential for a teen to experience intimidation, bullying, violence, or forced sexual activity is high. Communities that offer various enrichment programs, sports, edu-cation, or positive social experiences have lower numbers of teen parents.

Teens who live in neighborhoods with neighborhood unrest like vio-lence, gang activity, visible evidence of drug use or run-down buildings often live in fear, can be easily intimidated by, or suffer abuses from, peers or other people in the community. The combined lack of resources, employment, and housing contributes to teens being more likely to engage in, or be forced into, unprotected sexual activity that could lead to parenthood.

Being in the welfare or foster care system can also impact teen pregnancy. Teens who move from foster home to foster home, or who are locked into the welfare system as their only means of any financial support or other resources, are more likely to become teen parents.

Around the world there is evidence of people being segregated to certain neighborhoods by things like race, class, or religion. Where neighborhood segregation exists, those neighborhoods often lack adequate resources, employment opportunities, or housing, thus contributing to the likelihood of a teen becoming a parent.

There are many cultures globally who believe that teenage girls should be married and force girls to marry by a certain age. The age of the husband, however, can vary. These cultures also value children born to young or teen mothers and view teen parents as a normal aspect of society. Thus, teen girls who are married are often required to bear children for their husbands.

4. What problems do teen parents face?

Teen parents, like adult parents, face a variety of problems. However, teen parents are unique and have additional physical, social, emotional, or financial challenges. Although most of the existing research or evidence focuses on teen mothers, teen fathers or the teen parents together can be susceptible to issues, obstacles, or conflicts.

Teen Mothers

Teen mothers, overall, are least likely to seek timely medical care to confirm their pregnancy and start prenatal care. Many teen mothers do not have access to, or funds for, adequate prenatal care; issues or complications with a teen mother's pregnancy, or her baby, may go unrecognized or untreated. Teen mothers are also less likely to follow dietary or health maintenance recommendations and are more likely to smoke, have poor nutrition, or remain sexually active without using safe sex practices, or have a sexually transmitted disease (STD).

Although teenage girls begin to have regular menstrual periods and can become pregnant, their bodies continue to grow and mature throughout puberty and their teen years. Therefore, a girl's body may not physically be able to handle the burden of pregnancy if her growth and development are not completed. For example, a girl's pelvis might be too small or narrow to accommodate a growing baby within her uterus, or the birth canal could be too small or constricting to safely deliver a baby. In addition, a teen mother may have a small stature or body size that prevents her from carrying a baby comfortably.

During pregnancy, teen mothers are more susceptible to medical conditions associated with, or related to, the pregnancy. High blood pressure, or pregnancy-induced hypertension (PIH), is the most common complication found in teen mothers. Issues with blood pressure in teen mothers can quickly escalate into a worsening condition called preeclampsia where severely elevated blood pressures are accompanied by excess protein in the urine; swelling of the face, hands, and feet; excessive weight gain; persistent headaches; organ damage; and possibly seizures. The persistent high blood pressure in teen mothers causes decreased blood flow to the placenta which, in turn, deprives the baby of necessary nutrients for adequate growth.

A full-term pregnancy lasts about 40 weeks. Teen mothers, however, are more likely to go into labor prior to 40 weeks and deliver their babies prematurely. Babies born premature are often small and have a low birth weight, leaving them susceptible to a host of medical complications or injuries. Further, babies born premature and who survive the newborn period are still susceptible to developmental and behavioral issues, or health concerns, throughout childhood.

The challenges of being pregnant, or experiencing any of the complications of pregnancy, can cause a teen mother to be confined to bed rest or possibly be admitted to the hospital for several days or weeks. Many teen mothers are unable to attend school and may miss an entire year or must repeat a grade. Some teen mothers are forced to devote all their time to caring for the baby after delivery and may not return to school again. Therefore, teen mothers who do not complete their education, or ever attend college, are more likely to remain unemployed, be impoverished, or rely on publicly funded programs for housing and medical care for themselves and their baby. Employment opportunities for teen mothers, or women, without enough education or skills training, are few.

Because teen mothers often lack support or resources and may be faced with caring for an infant alone, stress is common. Stress can lead to teen mothers feeling overwhelmed, especially if adaptive coping skills have been developed. Persistent stress can lead to depression with many teen mothers reporting feeling sad or isolated.

Teen Fathers

Teen fathers face problems like teen mothers. Although teen fathers do not face the physical challenges of carrying or giving birth to a baby like teen mothers, they face unique social or financial problems. Teen fathers, however, are often overlooked when discussing teen pregnancy or parenthood; much of the existing focus of literature or research is based on the experiences of teen mothers. Teen fathers, then, are often the "forgotten partner."

Because teen mothers may be required to leave school and not work to care for a baby or child, teen fathers may need to also leave school to find work to provide for the needs of both the mother and the child. However, teen fathers often cannot find sustainable employment to allow them to support a family. Further, teen fathers who work often earn 10% to 15% less than adult working men. With the earning potential for teen fathers being poor, they are often inaccurately portrayed as lazy, uninvolved, or "deadbeats." Further, teen fathers are often stigmatized as reckless, deviant, or young men who lack any responsibility or direction. To the contrary, many teen fathers want to be involved in their child's life and often drop out of school to seek full-time employment to support their child. However, like teen mothers, employment opportunities for teen males are few, especially with insufficient or incomplete education.

Teen Parents

Teen parents also face problems as a couple. The relationship between the teen parents often changes, or is strained, when pregnancy occurs. Few couples marry, and social time that was used for dating, fun activities, or intimacy gets used for child care. The lack of finances or resources adds stress to the relationship, leading to an increased likelihood for arguments, breakups, or abuse. Both teen parents are susceptible to depression, anxiety, or feelings of inadequacy, being overwhelmed, guilt, or shame. Teen parents are also more likely to raise children who grow up to become teen parents themselves.

5. What are the possible long-term effects for a child born to teen parents?

Children of teen parents bear the greatest burden because of teen pregnancy. As such, those children are at significantly increased risk of long-term economic, social, and health effects. Thus, children of teen parents are at higher risk of growing up with emotional or educational problems. Because teen parents are more likely to live in poverty, they tend to have children that they are less likely to be able to support financially. Children of teen parents are more likely to endure long-term effects from infancy through adulthood.

Babies of teen parents are more likely to be born premature. As such, those babies of teen parents are more likely to be born with low or very low birth weight, which makes them more susceptible to, and more likely to develop, blindness, deafness, cerebral palsy at birth, mental illness beginning in childhood and extending into adulthood, and dyslexia or hyperactivity in childhood. Babies born to teen parents have more difficulty acquiring lifelong cognitive and language skills in addition to social and emotional skills like self-control or self-confidence. Therefore, children born to teen parents are less prepared to enter kindergarten.

Babies born to teen parents are also more likely to have less education. In addition, the children of teen parents are 50% more likely to repeat a grade or grades, and less likely to complete or graduate high school. Further, children of teen parents are more likely to perform poorly on standardized testing throughout their school years and achieve lower scores on the Preliminary Scholastic Aptitude Test (PSAT) or the Scholastic Aptitude Test (SAT) during high school years than their peers who were born to older parents.

Research supports that children of teen parents are more likely to live in poverty and experience more behavioral and health problems throughout childhood and adolescence. Thus, the children of teen parents are more likely to rely on publicly funded health care, and its restrictions or limitations, as their only source of health care or health insurance, health maintenance, or preventative care. Children of teen parents are more likely to suffer higher rates of abuse in multiple forms (e.g., verbal, physical, emotional, or sexual abuse) and neglect compared to children whose mothers had delayed childbearing.

Children of teen parents are more likely to not complete, fail, or drop out of high school. They are also more likely to remain unemployed, or underemployed, due to their lack of completed, formalized education. Children of teen parents are more likely to be incarcerated at some time during their adolescence or early adulthood. For example, sons of teen parents are 13% to 15% more likely to end up in prison compared to other boys or young men born to older adult parents. Daughters of teen parents are also 22% to 25% more likely to become teen mothers themselves.

6. What are the effects of teen pregnancy on a family?

Teen pregnancy is a life event that few families anticipate. However, the impact of teen pregnancy reaches far beyond the teen parents themselves.

There are emotional, economic, and social effects of teen pregnancy that affect a family in significant ways.

Emotional Factors

Parental reactions to a teen pregnancy range from denial and guilt to anger. Pregnant teens, however, share the same emotions. Therefore, the relationship between the teens and their parents, or their other family members, is often strained. Depending on the family's religious beliefs or social network, fear of being rejected or ostracized is a real possibility. Parents of pregnant teens may perceive the situation as a negative impression or reflection on themselves or their parenting skills. There is often a loss of trust between the parent and the teen after learning, and accepting, that the teen has been sexually active. There is also additional stress, worry, or anxiety as the parents focus on the safety of a teen mother due to a possible high-risk pregnancy. Further, pregnancy can cause a teen's parents to become depressed or withdrawn, thus impacting the family's overall emotional well-being. However, research demonstrates that many families reach a point of acceptance that leads the family to welcome the new baby and help the teen parents move forward with their life and education. As a teen parent accepts that they are now responsible for the life of a baby or a child, they seek guidance, parenting skills, and support or encouragement from their family members.

Economic Factors

A teen pregnancy can create a financial hardship, or obligation, for a family. Most times this financial responsibility falls on the family of a teen mother. Although the teen's parents may be employed or have adequate health insurance for themselves and the teen, many insurance plans deny maternity benefits to dependent children, thus increasing the financial burden to families of pregnant teens for prenatal care or delivery expenses. Further, following the baby's birth, the cost of the baby's health care and day-to-day living expenses (e.g., diapers, clothes, food) can have a significant impact on a family's budget or savings.

Social Factors

After revealing or discovering that a teen pregnancy exists, the family is faced with a critical decision about whether the teen will terminate the pregnancy, give the baby up for adoption, or keep the baby. Often a teen's parents, typically the mother of the pregnant teen, will step in to raise the baby of teen parents. The new grandmother often focuses her attention on the new baby and may have less time or energy to focus on her existing family, including her other children. The lack of focus or attention from the mother figure in the family can lead to, or promote, teen pregnancies in her other children, especially if the new grandmother is a single mother herself.

A teen pregnancy can also alter the goals or plans of the family. For example, a new baby of a teen parent may change the family's plans to travel, relocate, or vacation. A new baby can also impact the family's plans for retirement, ongoing education, or the education of other children, developing or maintaining new hobbies or exploring new interests. Care of the new baby or child, for a family, often becomes the priority.

7. What are the consequences of teen pregnancy for society?

Teen pregnancy affects more than the teen parents themselves; there is a significant impact on society or the communities at large that the teen parents belong to. Teen pregnancy is a global health problem. Regardless of where the teen pregnancy occurs, there are inherent needs for the children or parent's medical care and financial or social support. These supports, however, come at a cost for society.

One of the major consequences of teen pregnancy is that women or families will live at or below the poverty level. Most teen pregnancies occur to socioeconomically disadvantaged subpopulations that are typically in the lower strata of the community in developing countries. Women or girls within these subpopulations frequently lack adequate education or skills needed to sustain employment. In most cases, the biological father abandons the teen mother, and the baby becomes her sole responsibility. Hence, the mother ends up living in poverty and running the risk of imminent destitution. As teen pregnancies occur, more women or girls are likely to remain impoverished due to minimal opportunities for gainful employment or the inability to work because of child care.

Teen parents typically have low levels of education. Pregnant teens often perceive that caring for their baby or child is more important than obtaining or completing their education. Lack of education or skilled training prevents teens from securing stable employment, or keeps them unemployed, thus perpetuating the cycle of poverty. Researchers conclude that most teenage pregnancies end with education dropouts because of the fear of embarrassment, humiliation, and harassment from the fellow friends or peers. Illiteracy, then, is a real problem among teen mothers who do not complete their education.

Teen pregnancy poses significant financial burdens to society. The financial costs of teens who have babies are devastating. As the low-qualified mother cannot get a good job, she completely depends on welfare programs to overcome the impending financial distress. If teen parents are unable to be gainfully employed or remain employed, the society at large is often responsible for funding programs designed to assist teen parents or their child. For example, in the United States it is estimated that teen pregnancy can cost approximately 7 billion dollars annually due to lost tax revenue from teen parents who are not working, the cost to fund public assistance programs, the cost of health care for teen parents or their children, the maintenance of the foster care system, and criminal justice costs. Teen parents, typically, do not pay taxes, and the government must face a huge loss of revenue. Globally, teen girls who marry often do not work, reducing their future income or earnings by 9% to 15%. Thus, countries lose out on the annual income these young women would have earned over their lifetime.

Teen pregnancy leads to an increased number of single-parent homes and a breakup of the traditional family unit. Children raised in a single-parent environment are more likely to become teen parents themselves. Further, teens who marry are more likely to live in homes with threats of emotional or physical abuse and violence. Substance or alcohol abuse is also common in both families with a pregnant teen or within the homes of teens who marry. Teens who experience substance or alcohol abuse have diminished earning potential, again perpetuating a cycle of poverty. Most countries, developed and underdeveloped, consider teenage pregnancy a social stigma. Society usually considers teenage pregnancy a social dilemma, and young parents and their families must face humiliation and negative remarks from people.

8. What impact have media portrayals had on perceptions of teen pregnancy and parenthood?

The availability and types of media have exploded in the past decade (2010–2020). More than ever teens have an abundance of media, including books, magazines, music, the Internet and social media, movies, and television shows as sources of both entertainment and information. Teens are also the largest population using the various forms of media, especially electronic media like the Internet, social media, movies, and television. Teens represent a viable market for creators, producers, and advertisers for movies and television; programming specifically targeting teens is on the rise. Competition among advertisers, writers, or producers is ongoing with each trying to capture the largest share of the teen market. To ensure success, programming needs to stay cutting edge or interesting.

One area where programming has contended to push the envelope is teen pregnancy. The MTV franchise *16 & Pregnant* and its follow-up episodes and reality television shows like *Teen Mom* and its sequels or TLC's *Unexpected* attempt to explore the issues surrounding teen pregnancy by focusing on the lives of teen couples, their families, or their social circles. The theme among these shows is similar: to capture the various stages of each teen's pregnancy and the early weeks or months of parenthood. The teen couples are typically unprepared to have a child, so the parents, or grandparents and other relatives, of the teen mother or father are needed to assist the teen couple. Inevitably tension, stressors, or arguments ensue as all the different people involved clash or attempt to assert their opinions about the couple, their responsibilities, or their parenting. Consistent among all these shows, however, is that the teen couple is usually in close or regular contact and that abortion is never an option.

These shows have several commonalities. Each show displays a wide range of emotions. Like all teen parents, the cast members of the shows display the variety of emotions experienced by all teen parents. These include fear, anxiety, frustration, anger, happiness, excitement, or love. They also show how transformative teen pregnancy can be and demonstrate that teen pregnancy, and parenthood, has a significant impact on teen parents. The dramatic physical changes to the teen mothers' bodies during pregnancy are apparent, and the couple or mother often has complex health decisions to make both during and after pregnancy. There is also the element of deciding to stay pregnant and keep the baby while navigating how to reveal the pregnancy to friends or family.

Each show also demonstrates a noticeable change in each teen's identity and how society judges teen pregnancy and what is socially acceptable or unacceptable. There are often topics of who is a "bad" or "good" girl, or gossip about multiple sex partners and promiscuity. Despite this, the shows often portray that teen pregnancy is manageable. Consistent throughout all the shows about teen pregnancy is that the cast has some form of social, financial, or emotional support from family, their partner, or friends. There are also periods of humor interspersed with the issues or conflicts the teen couples face. Thus, the overtone that teen pregnancy is minimally different than one experienced by an adult couple, and therefore manageable, is apparent.

The shows, however, also make a point to emphasize that teen pregnancy is serious. The cast members of these shows acknowledge and reinforce that being a pregnant teen is not easy. Multiple instances are depicted where medical attention or visits to a health care practitioner, and medical decisions, are necessary. The reality of possible complications of a teen pregnancy are also portrayed.

Although these shows are unscripted, editing occurs to keep them within the specified limits of airtime for a television series. Because the content is selected by producers, an ongoing argument exists that these shows do not fully depict the realities of teen pregnancy. However, these shows are not intended to be a single source of information about safe sex or pregnancy prevention, hence a variety of real-life scenarios among the cast members are depicted. Thus, both positive and negative influences have been identified related to how media portrays teen pregnancy and parenthood.

Positive Influences

Most television shows about teen pregnancy and parenthood depict a positive outcome for the teen couple. The couple remains connected, involved, and supportive in each other's lives. There is also support, including emotional, social, and financial, from the teen's parents, grandparents, or friends. Despite the support from people in the teens' lives, the show highlights the difficulties the teen couple faces while trying to raise a child at a young age. The various emotions of being a teen parent are portrayed, including excitement, fear, love, anger, or happiness. Although a television show cannot be directly related to future teen behavior, a study done in 2014 after the end of *16 and Pregnant* found that there was a significant increase in the number of Internet searches for birth control and abortion among teens. Ironically, the rate of teen birth decreased by 5.7% during the year the research was conducted.

Negative Influences

Because teens are highly influenced by what they see or learn through various forms of media, there is growing concern that media portrayals of teen pregnancy glamorize teens being sexually active. A recent study found that teens are twice as likely to have sex or engage in sex acts if they see similar behaviors in the media. Cast or featured members of reality shows have been launched into instant fame or celebrity where their lives are photographed, followed, or reported in tabloids, television, or social media long after the television show has stopped airing. The celebrity status of the teen cast members conveys an idea that "cool" or "popular" teens are having sex and that teens having sex is normal. A subtle message is possibly conveyed by the media that teens should be sexually active as a sign of popularity, attractiveness, or maturity.

9. How can teen pregnancy be prevented?

The phenomenon of teen pregnancy is complex and multifactorial. Therefore, no single intervention will work to minimize or prevent teen pregnancy in the future. Because so many different factors influence teen pregnancy, a comprehensive approach is required; this includes parental involvement, targeted education, community resources, and health care services for both boys and girls.

Parental Involvement

Teens are influenced by the beliefs, values, ethics, behaviors, and examples of their parents from as early as infancy. Teens, then, are more likely to become pregnant if they were raised in an environment where teen pregnancy is supported or promoted or where parental actions steer a teen toward situations where teen pregnancy is more likely or inevitable. Therefore, parents, both as a couple or as a single-parent family, play an integral role in helping to prevent teen pregnancy.

Suggestions for how a parent or parents can play an active role in preventing teen pregnancy include the need for parents to strive to build and sustain a relationship based on love and acceptance, yet firm in discipline and rich in communication with their children and teens. Parents should also explore, and communicate, their own values and attitudes about sex. Teens are more likely to avoid sex or engage in sex acts if the expectations of the family are clear that teen pregnancy is discouraged, and that childbirth should be delayed until after marriage. Likewise, where permissible, parents should discourage early or teen marriage and emphasize a fulfilling life or education goals instead.

Parents should develop and promote open communication with children and continue that communication through teenage years, about sex and romantic relationships. It is never too early to begin conversations about sex, or discouraging sex, and these conversations should occur often. Further, these conversations should be free of any shame or embarrassment, so children or teens feel safe to ask questions.

Parents are also recommended to supervise and monitor their children's and teen's activities. Parents need to know what their children are doing, with whom, and where they are as often as possible. In addition, parents need to know who is in their child or teen's social circle. This includes knowing who their friends are, and the families of their friends, and who their child or teen spends their time with. Parents should also strive to know if the child or teen has any conflicts with peers or is being bullied by anyone in their environment.

Parents should set clear boundaries about dating. It is recommended that early, frequent, or steady dating is discouraged for both boys and girls, or at least until age 16. Teens should be encouraged to go out in groups, preferably with teens within a similar age range who the parents know. Further, parents need to set clear expectations about who a teen can date. Teens should be discouraged from dating older people; someone only one to two years older is the recommended age limit, if necessary, for dating.

Parents are advised to monitor a child or teen's use of media. Parents should be aware of what a teen is watching on television, or movies, reading in books or magazines, and the music they listen to. Internet use and social media need to be scrutinized. In addition, parents should emphasize the value of education and should support and encouraged teens to complete all formal education or skills training. Where appropriate, parents should communicate their expectations for college or advanced education or training. It is also suggested that parents encourage children and teens to develop other interests. Teens who continue to pursue activities like sports, music, art, dance, or clubs are more likely to both complete their formal education and delay engaging in sex or sex acts.

Targeted Education

Education can occur in any setting. However, teens should have specific topics explored and addressed, including abstinence from sex or sex acts to fully prevent pregnancy. There should also be information about all aspects of birth control including the various types available, how they work, the possible side effects, and how to obtain it. There also needs to be information about sex education, including safe sex practices, sexually transmitted infections (STIs), and emergency contraception.

The realities of pregnancy and childbirth, including potential complications, should be emphasized. There is also a need for education about child care or what is involved with raising a baby or child. This should include the proper and safe use of media and specific strategies for teens to maintain self-esteem, violence prevention, problem solving, and coping skills. Successful programs have been those that provide specific education for boys to avoid risky behaviors like fighting, gun use, gangs, etc.

Community Resources

The community a teen lives in can play an important role in preventing teen pregnancy. The community leaders should assess the surrounding environment and perform a comprehensive community assessment. This assessment should include the level of poverty within the community and its effects on families or teens. Adequate housing and the incidence of violence or drug use should also be considered. Most importantly, the community should determine what resources are available for teens, including schools, open or green space for sports or activities, community centers, or programs. Programs for teens that communities can develop include youth development programs that promote positive social behaviors and interactions among teens and within the community, healthy relationships, school achievements, and civic responsibility. These programs should also have abstinence education programs that promote abstinence from sex and sexual activity and emphasize the achievement of goals or dreams. Tutoring, or career counseling, helps to promote completing high school or acquiring additional skills or training for employment.

Health Care Services

Health care practitioners can provide medical or reproductive care or be sources of education or resources for teens. However, health care needs to be available and accessible for teens. Health care practitioners can advocate for the development of clinic-based family planning services located within communities to provide STI screenings, evaluations for appropriate birth control or contraception, abortion services or referral, or connections to social workers or other community resources. These services need to be confidential with easy access to birth control or contraception. There should also be the availability of referral for mental health services and advocacy for improved insurance coverage for teens.

Options for Pregnant Teens

10. What do I do if I decide to have an abortion?

For some women or girls, the decision whether to continue with an unplanned pregnancy or not may be a clear one. For others, the process is more difficult, making the decision about an unplanned pregnancy more complex. The decision about whether to have an abortion, however, is time sensitive and depending on how far along into the pregnancy (i.e., how many weeks gestation) a woman or girl is to determine how quickly she needs to make her decision. Further, location of abortion facilities, availability of getting an appointment, and the cost of the procedure also can have a significant impact on a woman's decision to have an abortion.

If a woman decides to have an abortion, there are some things she should do to both assist her in the decision-making process and to help her with her final decision. First, she should examine her beliefs and values related to pregnancy, parenting, and abortion. A woman needs to accept that she is the expert about her own life and she, therefore, knows what is best for her. She should examine what she needs, feels, or thinks about all the options available to her, including abortion. Further, she should explore those feelings related to *this* pregnancy, not ones she may or may not have in the future. She should consider what her goals, plans, and dreams are for the future and how a baby, or child, could impact achieving those goals. Above all, a woman should realize that, regardless of the decision, she has done her best to arrive at her decision and trust herself that she will make the best decision possible.

A woman will need to see her health care practitioner. Even with a positive home pregnancy test, a woman will need to confirm that she is, indeed, pregnant, and how far along the pregnancy is. With her health care practitioner, a woman can discuss her options and receive information. She should use this visit to ask questions and not feel pressured to decide about one option.

Regardless of her decision, a woman needs to understand her privacy rights. If the woman is an adult over the age of 18, she does not need to tell anyone about her decision to have an abortion, nor does she need familial or parental permission. However, in some instances where the woman is less than 18 years of age, she may be required to get a parent's, guardian's, or judge's permission before the procedure. This regulation varies state by state in the United States, and some have parental notification laws. It is important, then, to refer to the laws in each individual state.

A woman is advised to gather and use research or information carefully. There is a tremendous amount of information about abortion available, especially on the Internet. However, the information presented can be from sources that might be from the pro-choice or the pro-life movements that could influence the content that is provided. It is best, then, to discuss any questions or concerns with a health care practitioner.

Correct and accurate information will help a woman determine if a medical abortion is an option. There are different ways to complete an abortion, including a medical abortion. This specific method works best for women who are up to 10 weeks pregnant or about 70 days from the first day of their last menstrual period. A drug like mifepristone and/or misoprostol is used to complete the abortion and may be more suitable for some women. She should also research the option of a surgical abortion. A surgical abortion can be performed below 16 weeks gestation and might be a viable option for some women. However, after 16 weeks gestation other options may need to be considered.

There are multiple influences on whether a woman should have an abortion, so she should consider all factors. Aside from her personal beliefs and values, she should also consider her current financial situation, health status, family situation, and support network. A woman is encouraged to discuss her feelings with nonjudgmental friends, family, or support people. When facing a significant decision like whether to have an abortion, a woman should confide in people she trusts who can help her sort out her options and arrive at a decision. Counseling is also encouraged; the support, guidance, and referral of trained social workers or counselors can be invaluable to a woman, both before arriving at her decision to have an abortion or after. If there is no one in her immediate family or social network to help her, an unbiased social worker or counselor can be useful.

A woman needs to make a timely decision—20 to 24 weeks is often the latest allowable window where a woman could have an abortion. Therefore, a woman needs to make her decision by at least 20 weeks of gestation to avoid complications. She then needs to find a health care practitioner who performs abortions. A health care practitioner should be able to refer a woman to another provider who performs abortions if the health care practitioner does not perform the procedure themselves. There are various resources available on the Internet to help secure a reliable health care practitioner who safely performs the various types of abortions. It is important to also consider the distance that may be needed to travel to and from a health care practitioner for the procedure and any follow-up appointments, any mandatory state regulations regarding specified waiting periods before an abortion can be performed, and any costs that may be associated with the procedure.

Once an abortion is complete, it is important for a woman to prevent an unplanned pregnancy from happening again and consider birth control options for after the abortion. Options for birth control are often available immediately following the abortion (e.g., long-acting contraception, barrier methods). There are also several birth control options available for women that can be initiated at the follow-up visit after an abortion.

11. Are there different types of abortions, and how far into a pregnancy is each type available?

Although a miscarriage is an unintentional, often spontaneous loss of a pregnancy, an abortion is the deliberate termination of a pregnancy. Abortions are legal throughout most of the world, but laws surrounding them vary. For example, 60 countries currently, including most of Europe, allow abortion without any restrictions. Conversely, about 25 countries ban abortion totally with no exceptions. Abortion is legal in the United States during the first (i.e., 1 to 12 weeks gestation) and second (i.e., 12 to 24 weeks gestation) trimesters of pregnancy only, with most being performed during the first trimester. A few states permit an abortion up to the 24th week, but most prohibit abortions after the 20th week. In rare situations, a third trimester (i.e., 24 to 40 weeks) may be performed to save a mother's life. The type of abortion performed, then, is dependent on how far into the pregnancy (i.e., the weeks of gestation) a woman is. Abortion types include medical, vacuum aspiration, surgical, and induction.

Medical Abortion

A medical abortion is most successful when performed early in the first trimester, typically by 10 weeks gestation. A medical abortion involves a woman taking two different prescription medications: mifepristone and misoprostol. For a pregnancy to continue, progesterone is required; mifepristone blocks progesterone from the uterine lining, thereby causing the uterine lining to break down, thus preventing the ability to continue a pregnancy. Misoprostol causes the uterus to begin regular contractions to expel the fetus and other tissues from inside the uterus. Although medical abortions are generally safe and successful in most cases, there are some conditions that may make a medical abortion an unsuitable option for a woman. These include:

- An ectopic pregnancy (i.e., a pregnancy that implants outside the uterus).
- An allergy to mifepristone or misoprostol.
- The presence of a bleeding disorder or taking blood thinners (or anticoagulants).
- The presence of liver, kidney, or lung disease.
- An intrauterine device (IUD) in place.
- Long-term use of corticosteroid medications.

The procedure for a medical abortion requires a woman to obtain the two medications (either by prescription that is filled in a pharmacy or dispensed directly at a health care practitioner's office or clinic). The mifepristone is taken orally first. The misoprostol is taken orally a few hours, or up to 4 days, after the mifepristone. A woman can expect to begin to feel cramping and have possible heavy vaginal bleeding in about 1 to 4 hours after taking the dose of misoprostol. Other symptoms a woman may experience include:

- Nausea and vomiting.
- Diarrhea.
- Tiredness.
- Dizziness.
- Passing blood clots from the vagina.

Most women will pass the products of the pregnancy (i.e., fetus, placenta, uterine tissues) in about 4 to 6 hours after taking the pills. Some women may take up to 2 days to complete the abortion. A woman should rest and avoid work, school, exercise, sex, or strenuous activity for a few days after taking the pills.

A woman can typically expect to ovulate in about 3 weeks after taking the pills. Her period should start, then, within 4 to 6 weeks after taking the pills. Once ovulation resumes, a woman can get pregnant again, so having a method of birth control in place or not having sex is advised to prevent another unplanned pregnancy. If ovulation or menstrual periods do not resume, a follow-up appointment with a health care practitioner may be needed. A medical abortion should not interfere with a woman's ability to get pregnant in the future.

Vacuum Aspiration

Vacuum aspiration (also called suction aspiration or suction abortion) is one of the most common types of abortion performed, typically during the first trimester or early second trimester. This method is quick, usually painless, and successful. Some women need a vacuum aspiration if a medical abortion fails. Vacuum aspiration is often the preferred method of abortion if a woman has conditions like an abnormally shaped uterus, any blood-clotting disorders, a serious health problem or condition, or a pelvic infection.

Vacuum aspiration uses gentle suction to remove the contents of the uterus (i.e., the fetus and placenta). The procedure can be performed at a health care practitioner's office, clinic, or a hospital. After a woman is positioned on her back on an examination table with her legs in stirrups, a small cannula or tube is introduced through her cervix into her uterus. The suction is brief, lasting only about 5 to 10 minutes. The procedure is generally painless; however, a woman may feel some uterine cramping because the uterus contracts as the tissues are removed by the suction. Following the procedure, a woman often rests and is monitored for a few hours and then allowed to leave and go home. Some of the side effects a woman is instructed to watch out for include:

- Heavy bleeding or spotting.
- Persistent or worsening cramps.
- Nausea and/or vomiting.
- Worsening dizziness.
- Fever or unexplained abdominal pain.

Discomfort after the procedure is minimal, but aching or cramping can persist for 1 to 2 days. Over-the-counter (OTC) pain medications can often relieve the discomfort. A woman will typically ovulate about 3 weeks after the procedure and may have a menstrual period in about 4 to 6 weeks after the procedure. Women are advised to avoid sex until a method of birth control has been established (or at least 1 week after the procedure). A vacuum aspiration abortion should not affect a woman's ability to get pregnant in the future.

Surgical Abortion

Surgical abortion, also called a dilatation and evacuation (D&E), is not a common procedure. It is reserved for specific circumstances where an abortion is needed in the second trimester after the 14th week of gestation, typically for a woman who chooses to end a pregnancy because of a fetal abnormality or medical condition or when a woman delayed getting an abortion for too long.

Surgical abortion usually requires a health care practitioner who is skilled in performing this type of abortion. The procedure is usually performed in a clinic or hospital where sedation or anesthesia can be administered. Once a woman enters the operative area and is properly positioned for the procedure, the cervix is dilated or widened to permit entry of surgical instruments into the uterus. Specialized instruments are used to remove the fetus and the placenta; later suction or scraping of the uterine surface is used to remove any remaining tissues or uterine lining. The procedure lasts about 30 minutes to 1 hour. A woman will often recover and be monitored for a few hours after the procedure and be medicated for pain if needed. A woman usually goes home the same day but is instructed to observe for any increased bleeding, persistent or frequent cramping, nausea and/or vomiting, or fever and abdominal pain.

A woman is advised to avoid school, work, exercise, strenuous activity, or sex for 1 to 2 weeks after the procedure. Ovulation is likely to return in about 3 weeks after the procedure, and a woman can anticipate her menstrual period returning by 4 to 6 weeks after the procedure. A woman in usually advised to postpone resuming sexual activity until a form of birth control is in use if she wants to avoid another unplanned pregnancy. Women who desire pregnancy immediately after an abortion for fetal abnormality or medical condition may require genetic counseling or testing prior to attempting pregnancy again. However, a surgical abortion should not impact a woman's ability to become pregnant again.

Induction Abortion

An induction abortion is an alternative to a surgical abortion (or D&E); however, it is reserved for only unique circumstances where a pregnancy needs to be terminated after the 24th week of gestation or where a D&E is not possible to be performed.

An induction abortion is usually performed in a hospital, maternity, or birth center that offers monitored nursing and medical care for women. The procedure involves administering medications (orally, vaginally, or intravenously) that puts a woman into labor. Uterine contractions (i.e., labor) will follow that will dilate the cervix and eventually pass the fetus and placenta out of the uterus. Because the uterine contractions are progressive, strengthen in intensity and frequency, and painful, pain medications or specialized regional anesthesia (e.g., epidural medication or anesthesia) may be administered to make the induction more tolerable.

It can take several hours or a few days for an induction abortion to be completed. Careful monitoring and care from nurses and health care practitioners help minimize complications. Complications of an induction abortion can include pain, nausea and/vomiting, bleeding, cramping, diarrhea, chills, or other problems associated with labor or the delivery of a fetus.

A woman will need to recover for 1 to 2 days after an induction abortion. She will need to avoid school, work, strenuous activity, exercise, and sex for about 2 to 6 weeks after the procedure. For a woman who has an induction abortion for fetal abnormalities or medical conditions, she may require further genetic testing or counseling prior to becoming pregnant again. Women who wish to avoid another unplanned pregnancy will need to have a form of birth control in use prior to resuming sexual activity.

12. What are the costs associated with an abortion?

Like any medical or surgical procedure, abortions have associated costs. Those costs, however, can vary. In the United States, the cost of an abortion is dependent on multiple factors like location, type of facility or procedure performed, insurance coverage, and current health policy.

Location

The state a woman lives in can have a significant impact on abortion costs. For example, states where abortion laws are the most restrictive

often have the highest abortion costs compared to states with more supportive laws in favor of abortion. Clinics tend to be funded differently
than private health care practitioner offices or hospitals, so costs could be
higher in smaller, private centers to cover both the cost of the procedure
and the facility's additional expenses like staff payroll, supplies, the lease,
or security. It is not uncommon, then, for costs to vary between clinics
or practices within the same city or within the same state. Places where
abortions can be performed may be few or remote in certain areas, adding
an extra travel expense for women to get to and from them.

Type of Facility

Where an abortion takes place can also impact the costs associated with
the procedure. Clinics often receive state and federal funding, so they
may be able to provide sliding scale payment systems, especially in areas
where a large portion of the community served is poor, has low income,
or are unable to pay (like teens). Health care practitioners' offices are
funded or maintained by the revenue generated from the patient volume
within the practice. Because these types of practices have significant
overhead and additional fees associated with owning and managing a
practice, abortion costs could also be high. Hospitals, however, are often
the most expensive places to have an abortion since multiple costs and
fees are inherent within a hospital. Hospitals are utilized for complicated abortions or those further along in the second trimester because
additional equipment, monitoring, and personnel are required, thus
increasing cost.

Type of Abortion

The type of abortion a woman has is determined by how far along into the
pregnancy she is. However, the different types of abortions have fluctuating costs based on what is required to complete the procedure (see table,
Average Cost of Abortion by Type). Medical abortions, at present, are the
most cost effective or inexpensive. The procedure only requires a brief visit
with a health care practitioner and the cost of the two pills. Some centers
are modernizing their processes for medical abortion and use telehealth
or virtual visits to minimize costs and expedite a woman's access to the
medications.

Vacuum aspiration abortions are moderately priced higher compared to
a medical abortion. Vacuum aspiration requires the use of a center, facility, or health care practitioner's office that has specialized instruments and

Average Cost of Abortion by Type

Type of Abortion	Mean Cost	Cost Range	Comments
Medical abortion	$535	$75–$1,600 or higher	
Vacuum aspiration abortion	$500	$400–$1,000	
Surgical abortion (i.e., D&E)	Not applicable	$500–$3,000 or higher	Additional costs for hospital stay, anesthesia services, personnel, etc.

equipment, and the personnel, to safely perform the procedure. A surgical abortion (i.e., a D&E), in contrast, is the most expensive. The fees associated with a hospital stay, the use of an operating room and anesthesia services, plus the various personnel needed to complete the procedure safely incur significant costs. Insurance coverage for any abortion procedure, however, remains variable, unreliable, and inconsistent.

Insurance Coverage

Women with health insurance can face a significant financial burden trying to navigate the cost of an abortion if needed. Having health insurance is also not a guarantee that an abortion will be covered. Although some organizations assist with funding centers to help women obtain an abortion, there are few additional resources available outside of any government funding for certain clinics. Medicaid, for example, only covers abortion services in some circumstances, but that coverage varies state by state.

Insurance regulations change and vary for each insurance company. Some plans cover abortion as a gynecologic procedure or part of routine care. However, these plans are few and often have restrictive or defined parameters for coverage (e.g., the health care practitioner or the facility used must be in network). Some states restrict abortion coverage in insurance plans offered under the current health exchange or restrict abortions for public employees covered under a group plan. Despite recent federal health care reform, some states also limit coverage for abortion under private insurance. Abortions, then, are constantly under scrutiny, and debate in the political arena and the values, beliefs, and decisions of current elected officials determine the funding of abortions in both public programs and private insurance.

Health Care Policy

Elected officials are charged with carefully using state or federal funds and determine funding for, and costs of, health care services in their communities. It is rare that any federal, state, or private insurance plan covers an abortion entirely. States, then, determine what programs to fund, and some states restrict or regulate abortion, thus making access to them difficult for women. However, making access to safe abortion services difficult only means women must go to greater lengths to have one. Ironically, the greatest restrictions and regulation often impact the communities where abortion services and health care are most needed (i.e., low income or impoverished areas). The future of abortion, especially in the United States with a volatile political climate surrounding abortion since its legalization, always remains uncertain.

13. What are the possible complications of an abortion?

Abortions performed in the United States and other developed nations are generally safe. Complications from abortions are low and occur in only 1 out of every 250 to 1,000 vacuum aspiration–type abortions and only 1 out of 1,000 medical abortions. However, complications can occur in both medical and surgical-type abortions.

Medical Abortion

Complications from a medical abortion are extremely rare, especially if the abortion is completed early (i.e., less than 49 days). The rate of complications increases to 4% between days 50 to 56 and about 9% between days 57 to 63. The most common complication that may occur with a medical abortion is abortion failure. Despite the effectiveness of mifepristone and misoprostol, there may be an occasion where the drugs do not work, and the pregnancy continues. Typically, a woman will report little to no bleeding or cramping after taking both medications and may continue reporting symptoms of pregnancy. A health care practitioner will likely perform a physical examination and an ultrasound scan of the uterus to determine if a woman is still pregnant. If a continuing pregnancy is found, and depending on how far into the pregnancy a woman is when a continuing pregnancy is discovered, a vacuum aspiration abortion may be needed to complete the procedure.

A rare complication with a medical abortion is infection. The medications associated with a medical abortion do not cause an infection.

However, the process of emptying the uterus exposes the uterus and other structures within the reproductive tract to any pathogens that might be present in the vagina or on the cervix. If a woman has an undiagnosed sexually transmitted infection (STI), her risk of infection increases. Signs and symptoms of infection include persistent abdominal pain, fever, nausea, and vomiting, foul-smelling or heavy vaginal discharge, weakness, and headache. Infections can be serious and can progress rapidly without prompt treatment. A health care practitioner will perform a thorough physical examination and possibly blood tests to confirm a diagnosis. If the infection is severe, a woman may require hospitalization. Antibiotics are a common treatment and follow-up is needed to ensure the infection has resolved.

Surgical Abortion

The most common type of surgical abortion performed is the vacuum aspiration. Although complications are rare with this procedure, a possible complication is a uterine perforation. The instruments used in the abortion procedure, like any other gynecologic surgery or procedure performed within or around the uterus, can puncture the uterine wall. The degree of severity depends on how large the perforation is. Women may experience abdominal pain, mild to heavy vaginal bleeding, or fever. Most perforations resolve on their own but larger perforations may require surgery to repair them.

The uterus is exposed to all the microorganisms present in the vagina or on the cervix when the cervix is dilated, and instruments are introduced into the uterus. The risk of infection increases if a sexually transmitted infection (STI) is present. A woman may experience persistent abdominal pain, fever, nausea, and vomiting, foul-smelling or heavy vaginal discharge, weakness, and headache. Infections can be serious and can progress rapidly without prompt treatment. A health care practitioner will perform a thorough physical examination and possibly blood tests to confirm a diagnosis. If the infection is severe, a woman may require hospitalization. Antibiotics are a common treatment and follow-up is needed to ensure the infection has resolved.

Like any other gynecologic procedure or surgery, the instruments used to complete a vacuum aspiration–type abortion can cause injuries to the reproductive tract like tears or lacerations to the cervix or the walls of the vagina. The degree of severity depends on how large or deep the tear or laceration may be, or if it occurs near any blood vessels. A woman may notice persistent spotting or a trickling of blood from the vagina along with discomfort in the vaginal area. Injuries to the reproductive tract can often be diagnosed by direct visualization of the vagina or cervix by a health care practitioner during a pelvic examination. Most injuries are superficial and heal on their own; more extensive injuries will require sutures (i.e., stitches) to promote closure of the area and eventual healing.

Bleeding can occur at any time during a vacuum aspiration–type abortion. The placenta and uterus are vascular structures so manipulation, especially with surgical instruments or gentle suction, can cause bleeding. Mild, light bleeding is common. Heavy, persistent, or uncontrolled bleeding (i.e., hemorrhage) is a medical emergency that requires immediate intervention.

Common to any kind of abortion is regret. Although not a typical complication in the medical or surgical domain that affects the functioning of the body, regret is real and can cause a host of emotional symptoms like depression, anxiety, or fear. Abortion is permanent, and once the procedure is completed there is no way to reverse it.

14. Can I get an abortion without telling my parents?

Although many teens faced with an unintended pregnancy choose to involve their parents, there are more who choose not to. Some teens cannot involve their parents, have no access to their parents, are too afraid or embarrassed to tell their parents, or face threats of violence in their home if an unintended pregnancy is discovered.

Confidentiality in medical treatments, including treatments related to sexual or reproductive health, is a protected constitutional right to privacy for teens. Therefore, if a teen is less than 18 years of age, she may not have to tell her parent(s) to obtain an abortion. However, individual states have created laws that have redefined whether a teen needs a parent's permission to obtain an abortion or not.

Some states do not have any laws about notifying parents or getting their permission to obtain an abortion. However, some states mandate that teens must get permission from their parent, older family member, or guardian to obtain an abortion. Other states do not require permission, but a teen's parent(s) will be notified that a teen is obtaining an abortion. In rare cases, a judge may be able to grant permission for a teen to obtain an abortion without notifying either parent.

As recent as June 2019, most states in the United States (i.e., 37) have some form of legislation that requires parental involvement in a minor's decision to have an abortion. In addition:

- 21 states require only parental consent; 3 of those states (i.e., Kansas, Mississippi, and North Dakota) require both parents' consent.

- 5 states require both parental notification that a teen is seeking to obtain an abortion and their consent for the teen to have the procedure performed.
- 7 states permit a minor to obtain an abortion if a grandparent or other adult relative is involved in the decision.

Some teens have open communication with their parents that is determined by the quality of the relationship between the teen and the parent. However, even teens with supportive relationships with parents still struggle with the fear, disappointment, and potential disconnection from their families if they tell their parents or have them involved. Indeed, parental involvement can delay a teen's access to abortion care or services. Although parents cannot force a teen to have an abortion, the various laws requiring parental involvement have led teens to go to states where parental involvement laws are less restrictive.

Individual state laws can be confusing and difficult to navigate. Several reliable resources are available on the Internet that help explain state laws and requirements more clearly (e.g., the Guttmacher Institute). However, health care practitioners and clinics or facilities are very aware of the laws surrounding abortion in the state where they practice and are valuable resources to teens. They can also discuss options with teens and assist teens with tips or advice on talking with parents about abortion.

Teens deserve the right to access any reproductive or sexual health services needed, including abortion care. Abortion providers will only perform the procedure on a woman who has made an informed decision to have an abortion freely. Hence, advocates for women's health are working to minimize harmful parental involvement restrictions that can put a teen's health and well-being at risk and secure legislation to protect women's, and girls', access to abortion services. Specifically, advocates are seeking targeted legislation that considers teens and protects their access to safe, legal, and affordable abortion care.

15. How does the adoption process work?

The legal process of adoption is what transfers the permanent parent-child relationship from one party to another. Adoption provides the adoptive parents the rights and responsibilities of a legal parent and makes the child a legal member of the family.

For both parents considering placing their child for adoption, the legal requirements can seem overwhelming and confusing. Several laws dictate the process of adoption, which varies state by state. Understanding the law surrounding adoption helps a teen parent or couple make the best decision possible. Because adoption laws differ state by state, the adoption process can vary based on where the birth parents and adoptive parents live. The adoption process is different for every mother or family depending on what she needs during pregnancy and what she wants her adoption plan to be.

The process for initiating adoption follows a basic pathway. First, a woman or couple needs to determine if adoption is the right option. This is likely the biggest and hardest decision a teen parent can make, so considering adoption options is important. Every woman's situation is different, and each woman knows what is right for her and her baby. A health care practitioner can help a teen mother, or couple, navigate their options to arrive at a decision.

With any adoption, the mother oversees the adoption plan and determines how to go about putting her baby up for adoption in a way that is comfortable for her. Working with a lawyer, social worker, or adoption professional (that a social worker can help secure) is essential. An adoption professional will work closely with a mother or teen family to ensure their wishes for the adoption are fulfilled. The adoption professional will help a teen family navigate if they want to have any contact or communication with the baby, and how often, before, during, and after the delivery of the baby. Therefore, understanding the adoption process is a primary step in the adoption process. An adoption professional can help a teen mother or couple to plan and discuss their needs during pregnancy. Adoption professionals are resources for a teen mother or couple to answer questions and navigate the adoption process.

An adoption professional will also assist a teen parent or couple to determine how the adoption process will continue, including a plan for the labor and delivery stay and how, or if, the potential adoptive parents will be involved. The adoption professional will assist the mother with securing any additional resources she may need like housing, food, maternity clothes, or other items needed for the pregnancy or delivery.

There are different options a teen parent can have with the adoptive family. The teen mother determines what kind of relationship with the adoptive parents she thinks would work best for her. The adoption professional finds families who are willing to collaborate with the teen mother to meet her wishes. A pregnant teen opting for adoption does not have to choose the adoptive family for her baby, but she can participate in choosing the family who will adopt her child. Information about each prospective family will be sent to the mother to review and decide based on their profiles. Communication with prospective families can be arranged through the adoption professional.

The adoption professional will help provide any support or other resources needed, or coordinate having the potential adoptive family present for the birth or immediately after depending on the mother's preference. The state the birth mother lives in determines when she must relinquish her baby to the adoptive parents.

16. Are there different types of adoption?

There are several types of adoption available to pregnant teens. In general, adoptions are considered closed or open type.

Closed adoption is one where no identifying information about the birth family or the adoptive family is shared between the two, and there is no contact between the two families. The adoptive family receives minimal information about the child and the birth family. The birth mother will also receive few details about the family adopting the baby. Depending on the state where the adoption takes place, the adoption records may be sealed. Local law, further, may also determine if those records are available to an adopted child when they reach a certain age (e.g., 18).

Open adoption allows for some form of contact or association between the birth parents, the adoptive parents, and the adopted child. The degree of contact ranges from pictures or letter sharing regularly to phone calls or contact through a liaison or intermediary. In some cases, adoptive parents allow full, regular contact between the adopted child and the birth family.

Within the adoption system there are several ways to adopt a child. These options are also available to teen parents who may be looking for safe ways to place their child up for adoption. These options include:

- *Foster care.* Parents who cannot care for their child (or children) themselves or learn that they cannot bear the burden of raising a child, can opt to put their child in foster care. Foster care is meant to be temporary, but for some children foster care can lead to adoption. When foster care evolves into adoption, the birth parent(s) typically give up their paternal rights to the child.
- *Foster care to adoption.* Some children are placed into a foster home with the understanding that, over time, the child will eventually

become eligible to be adopted. The foster family has an option to adopt the child themselves and bring the child into their family.

- *Infant adoption.* There are many families who are seeking to adopt an infant. Indeed, there are more families waiting to adopt a baby than there are babies available for adoption. Parents looking to adopt an infant will often use an intermediary like a lawyer, physician, or facilitator to make an introduction to a mother who is willing to give her baby up for adoption rather than go through an adoption agency. Known as an *independent adoption*, this is a direct arrangement between the birth mother and father and the adoptive parents. However, the laws surrounding this type of adoption vary from state to state.

- *Adoption through an agency.* Adoption agencies can be public or private and are regulated by the state. Therefore, they must be licensed to place children with prospective adoptive parents. Public adoption agencies typically handle children who are, for example, wards of the state, abandoned, orphaned, abused, or older in age.

- *Private adoption agencies.* Private adoption agencies are often run by charities or social service organizations. These agencies will typically place children who have been brought to the agency by parents or expectant parents seeking to give their child up for adoption.

- *Adoption through identification.* A potential adoptive family may find a mother who wants to put her baby or child up for adoption. If the birth family agrees to the adoption, then both families complete the adoption process through an adoption agency. The advantage to this process is that both the birth family and the adoptive family select each other, and the adoptive family does not have to be on a waiting list indefinitely in the hope of finding a child or baby.

- *International adoption.* This is the most complicated type of adoption and one that is more common with families who are seeking to adopt as opposed to families who are looking to give their child up for adoption. To adopt a child or baby who is a citizen of a foreign country, there are multiple laws in the state where the adoptive parents live as well as laws from the home country of the child or baby to abide by. Adoptive parents have legal processes to go through, including obtaining a visa for the child to be adopted to come to the United States. As of 2008, international adoptions are regulated through the Hague Adoption Convention. This treaty provides U.S. federal government oversight of domestic adoption agencies and international adoption policies to protect children, birth parents, and adoptive parents from unethical adoption practices.

17. If I decide to keep my baby, what do I need to provide my child with once it's born?

A baby, and later a child, has multiple needs after it is born. A baby is completely dependent on its parents for all its immediate needs. As the baby grows and enters different age groups, their needs change and often the cost of meeting those needs increases.

Raising a child is expensive. Certain expenses become necessary, while others occur because they need to be continually replaced. Cost, however, varies depending on the location where one lives; in the United States, the northeast and urban areas of the western regions are the most expensive places to raise children. According the U.S. Department of Agriculture (USDA), the average yearly cost to raise a child from birth to age 2 is about $12,680. That cost increases slightly to $12,730 for a child age 3 to 5 and further increases to $13,180 by age 9. By the time a child reaches age 15 to 17, the annual cost rises to $13,900. Single-parent families making less than $59,200 per year can expect to spend about $9,000 per year to raise an infant and over $10,000 per year to raise a child by age 15.

Regardless of age, a baby or child will require housing. Often the largest expense for parents, children need a home that provides shelter within a safe environment. In the United States adequate shelter includes running water, plumbing, and appropriate temperature control like heating.

All human beings require nutritious food to survive, grow, and develop. Although infants can receive nourishment from breastfeeding or commercial infant formula for the first year of life, eventually a child requires a variety of foods to provide nutrition. A child also needs to eat regularly throughout the day (i.e., three meals per day and healthy snacks). Children also need appropriate clothing to accommodate the climate they live in. However, children grow and change rapidly during the first two decades of life, thus making the need for clothing a frequently recurring expense

Babies need to be evaluated by a health care practitioner at regular intervals to assess for adequate growth, achievement of developmental milestones, and to receive immunizations to prevent diseases. Children also require at least a yearly evaluation of their growth and development, updated immunizations, and most often episodic care or treatment for illness or injuries. Although publicly funded health care is available, costs for health care can be significant for a parent or family. Further, if a teen parent continues their education or opts to work, the child will need to be watched and cared for by a responsible adult. Regular, ongoing child care can be costly.

Children require schooling and education from as early as preschool through high school. Although there is usually a public school system maintained by the community and local government for free education of children, there are expenses associated with school, including supplies, books, or other school-related activities. Children will also need to get from place to place, like school or activities, safely. When walking to each destination is not an option, parents need to rely on public transportation or purchasing their own private vehicle.

Beyond the physical things a child needs, they also require intangible things that are equally important. For example, children need safety and security, including within their home, their community, and in their school. They also require protection from harm, including harmful influences, factors, or substances in their home, environment, and community. Most importantly, children need love and emotional support from their parents and other family members who serve as positive role models.

18. What resources are available if I decide to keep the baby?

Teen parents attempt to raise a healthy child while potentially trying to navigate school, work, their future, and teenage life. There are different state or federal programs, or resources, available to aid teens who decide to keep their baby. A social worker, counselor, or health care practitioner can assist teens to navigate the various programs and resources and their individual application processes.

Title IX is a federal law that protects teen parents by prohibiting discrimination, including for pregnant teens, in schools. Title IX requires schools to excuse absences for pregnancy, childbirth, or related conditions. It provides teen mothers the opportunity to stay in school and complete their education. It requires schools to provide pregnant students with the same services and accommodations equal to those provided to nonpregnant students (e.g., home schooling, tutoring, independent study) or attend a separate program for pregnant and parenting students if they wish.

Women, Infants, and Children Nutrition Assistance, or WIC, is a special supplemental nutrition program for qualifying low-income women and their babies. To access WIC, a woman must be pregnant or breastfeeding at the time of the application. Women who gave birth and not breastfeeding, children up to age 5, or infants less than a year old can also access the program to receive benefits. Mothers receive vouchers (or, in some states, an electronic debit card) that allow her to purchase nutritious food. WIC participants also have access to nutrition education and referrals to other social service programs, access to immunization and health screenings, breastfeeding counseling, and substance abuse referrals if needed.

The Supplemental Nutrition Assistance Program (SNAP), or also commonly known as "food stamps," provides a monthly supplement for women or families to purchase a wide variety of nutritious food, including fresh fruit and vegetables. To obtain SNAP benefits, certain eligibility requirements need to be met. Unlike WIC, this is specifically designed to assist women, children, or infants during important development stages. SNAP assists people, including men, across the life span. It may be possible for teen mothers to receive both SNAP and WIC benefits.

The Temporary Assistance for Needy Families (TANF) is a cash assistance program that helps low-income families afford food, housing, and child care expenses. Parents or caretakers who cannot afford to pay for their household's basic needs may apply for benefits and, during the application process, may also discover they qualify for other government assistance programs. The TANF program, however, is designed to be short term and to assist families to work toward self-sufficiency by providing training or resources needed to secure future employment opportunities. In some states TANF programs may provide additional benefits like child care assistance, help with obtaining a GED (graduate equivalency diploma), or vocational training.

Medicaid is the U.S. public health insurance program that provides health care coverage to low-income families or individuals. It covers visits to a health care practitioner, hospital stays, long-term medical care, and other related costs. It is a jointly funded program between the federal government and the individual states. It is operated at the state level, so coverage provided, and administration of the program, varies greatly from state to state. Medicaid is only available to individuals or families who meet specific income requirements and are U.S. citizens, permanent residents, or legal immigrants. In contrast, the Children's Health Insurance Program (CHIP) provides low-cost health coverage to children in families that earn too much money to qualify for Medicaid but not enough to pay for private insurance. Each state offers CHIP coverage and works with its Medicaid program to insure adequate coverage for children. In some states CHIP covers pregnant women.

19. What financial assistance is available to teen mothers and their children?

There are several financial assistance programs available to single parents, including teen mothers. What is important to remember is that most of the programs are managed by each individual state; benefits and programs vary from state to state and may vary from county to county within each state. Further, most of the programs are administered through each state's individual welfare programs. Because welfare programs are based on income, teen mothers need to be aware of the qualifying criteria for welfare assistance within the state they live in. For example, in many states a teen mother who still lives at home with her parents may fall under her parents' income structure and therefore not qualify for any assistance programs.

The financial assistance programs are designed to provide resources and help for specific needs. For example, resource programs like WIC, SNAP, or TANF address the need for food to feed a family through their voucher or electronic debit card system. Financial assistance programs, typically, do not dispense cash or checks directly to a teen mother; instead, funds are paid directly to specific areas (e.g., child care providers, landlords) or are provided as credit for purchases.

There are some well-known examples of financial assistance programs for teen mothers. These include grants for low-income single parents for housing, child care, or scholarships. Single teen mothers who work often qualify for federal tax credits or breaks like the Earned Income Tax Credit, which is a benefit for working people with a low to moderate income. In addition, the Child Tax Credit gives up to $2,000 for each child living with a qualifying single parent. The Additional Child Tax Credit gives single parents a payment for any additional children they may have in the home if no tax is owed. If a teen mother finishes high school and seeks to go back to college for a bachelor's degree, the U.S. Department of Education offers Pell grants. Qualifying single mothers can earn up to $6,000 to be used at any participating school. Unlike a loan, the money from a Pell grant does not need to be repaid.

The U.S. Department of Agriculture (USDA) offers free lunch (and sometimes breakfast depending on the school system and the area a mother lives in) through the National School Lunch Program for school-aged children, even during the summer months. There is also the Emergency Food Assistance Program (TEFAP), where the USDA buys emergency food and ships it directly to states to distribute within their food pantries or directly to low-income people who qualify for food assistance.

The Housing Choice program, formerly known as "Section 8," is funded by the U.S. Department of Housing and Urban Development (HUD) and offers low-income mothers rental housing. There is also the Low Income Home Energy Assistance Program (LIHEAP) and the Weatherization Assistance Program, which helps qualifying candidates, including single mothers, to pay utility bills. These programs also offer incentives to help insulate homes or correct defects in homes to help reduce energy costs.

The state Department of Education offers affordable child care to low-income families while the parent is working, attending school, or a training program through the *Child Care Assistance Program (CCAP)*. A single mother pays a small portion of the overall cost of child care based on her income. Head Start programs are free child care programs that promote a child's education and development. These programs are state run and use federal funds to prepare children up to age 5 for school.

Beside federal and state programs, a variety of religious organizations and not-for-profit charities also offer programs to help teen mothers. These organizations also support programs like food pantries, shelters, or clothing resources to assist families in need. The services of these organizations are often like government programs, but they are funded through philanthropy, donations, or fund-raising activities. Because these organizations secure their own funds, they often have less restrictive qualifying criteria for teen mothers to receive assistance.

20. What do I do if I keep the baby and then I can't handle things anymore?

Raising a baby can be stressful. Feeling overwhelmed is common; it can range from something momentary like "I'm fed up" to more persistent, profound feelings of not being fit to be a parent or handle day-to-day life. There are multiple reasons that can contribute to teen parents feeling overwhelmed, including difficulty meeting a baby's needs, financial burdens, lack of support or resources, or addictions. When caring for a baby becomes overwhelming, teen parents may not be aware of the options available to them. The primary concern is the safety of the baby and the teen parents. Teen parents should know that there are services and resources to help them if caring for a baby becomes too much to handle.

Each state in the United States has some form of Safe Haven statutes. Safe Haven allows parents of any age to leave an unharmed newborn at designated safe places like hospitals, police stations, or fire stations without the fear of criminal charges for abandonment. A baby can be left without the parent having to disclose their identity or answering questions. Most states, however, limit the age of an infant who can be left at a Safe Haven location; many require the infant to be 72 hours old or younger, but some will accept an infant up to 1 month of age. After leaving the infant, the parent in most cases has up to 30 days to get their baby back. The Safe Haven locations ensure the baby's safety and prevent babies from being abandoned in an unsafe environment or condition.

Child or infant abandonment is illegal in the United States. Abandonment refers to a parent's choice to willfully withhold physical, emotional, and financial support from a minor child. To prevent infants or children from being abandoned, there are several resources for teen parents. One of the first people a teen should turn to is a trusted adult family member or friend. A teen can also reach out to a teacher, school counselor, health care practitioner, or social worker. Any professional can assist a teen parent to access resources or develop a plan to care for the baby.

Each state has its own child welfare service. These services can be contacted to help take a child out of an unsafe environment and placed into an alternative, safer arrangement. The foster care system strives to keep infants and families together. Infants or children may be placed with other relatives or a responsible family that is able to care for them temporarily. These agencies work with teen parents to provide any needed resources, education, or support to make them more effective parents or reunite them with their baby.

If a teen parent continues to find themselves unable or unwilling to care for their baby, a teen parent has the option to put their baby up for adoption. The same professionals who assist with foster care can also refer a teen to the right resources to explore adoption. Social workers are an invaluable resource for information and support to teens and can help develop a plan that will best fit the needs of the parent and baby.

Pregnancy, Delivery, and Medical Concerns for Teens

21. How do the menstrual cycle and conception work?

A woman's monthly period, or the predictable days of vaginal bleeding that occurs about the same time each month, is called her menstruation. This monthly bleeding is the shedding or sloughing of the lining of the uterus when conception (or pregnancy) does not occur. Most menstrual periods last 3 to 5 days. The menstrual cycle encompasses all the different hormonal and physical changes a woman's body goes through from the first day of one month's menstrual bleeding (i.e., the first day of bleeding) to the first day of the next month's menstrual bleeding. However, the menstrual cycle is more than just the actual menstrual period; it is an intricate balance of hormones that work together in a cyclical fashion to promote ovulation, fertilization, or potential pregnancy.

Most women can accurately count the days from the beginning of one period to the beginning of the next. Typical menstrual cycles range from 21 to 35 days, with the average menstrual cycle lasting 28 days. During the menstrual cycle, important body chemicals called hormones rise and fall at different points to prepare a woman's body for pregnancy. This rise and fall of specific hormones are what regulates, or controls, the menstrual cycle.

At the beginning of the menstrual cycle, levels of the key female hormone, estrogen, begin to rise. Estrogen is produced in the ovaries, adrenal glands, and fat tissue. The rise of a stimulating hormone called luteinizing hormone causes estrogen to be produced in those specific areas, thereby increasing the level of estrogen in the bloodstream. As estrogen levels rise, the lining of the uterus responds and begins to grow and thicken. While the uterine lining is growing, one of a woman's ovaries begins to mature an egg, or ovum. By about day 14 or 15 of a typical 28-day menstrual cycle, the egg is released from the ovary, hence the term "ovulation." Women with varying, or unpredictable, menstrual cycles, in contrast, may ovulate before or after day 14. It is within the 2 to 3 days prior to ovulation, the day of ovulation, or 1 to 2 days immediately following ovulation that a woman is most likely to become pregnant.

After the egg leaves the ovary, it travels down the fallopian tube toward the uterus. Hormone levels continue to rise, and the thickened uterine lining is maintained. The surge of hormones changes a woman's natural cervical mucus to become thinner and more slippery to allow sperm to travel easily up into the uterus to meet the egg for fertilization. If a woman has sex during this time, and semen is ejaculated into the vagina, the sperm cells have a convenient path into the uterus to unite with the egg that was released. When the sperm and egg unite, fertilization, or conception, occurs. The fertilized egg continues traveling down the fallopian tube toward the uterus. The thickened uterine lining is an ideal place for the fertilized egg to embed for nourishment as it continues to develop at a rapid pace.

22. How can I tell if I'm pregnant?

Following conception, a woman may begin to experience the signs or symptoms that she is pregnant as early as 10 days to 2 weeks. However, each woman is different, and each woman experiences the signs and symptoms of pregnancy at different times. The signs and symptoms of pregnancy can be broken down into three different categories: presumptive symptoms, probable signs, and definitive signs.

Presumptive Symptoms

Presumptive signs and symptoms of pregnancy are suggestive that a woman may be pregnant but could also indicate the presence of another medical condition. Typically, presumptive signs and symptoms of pregnancy occur early (about 3 to 8 weeks after conception) and are often more subjective (i.e., the symptoms a woman experiences are ones that she can feel or describe) than other signs or symptoms. Presumptive signs and symptoms of pregnancy include, but are not limited to:

- Amenorrhea—the absence of, or a missed menstrual period.
- Nausea with or without vomiting.
- Fatigue.
- Poor sleep.
- Back pain.
- Constipation.
- Food cravings or aversions.
- Heartburn.
- Nasal congestion.
- Shortness of breath.
- Lightheadedness.
- Headaches.
- Mood swings or changes.
- Frequent urination.
- Breast tenderness, enlargement, or tingling.

Probable Signs

Probable signs of pregnancy are those that are noticeable by a health care practitioner during a physical examination. These signs, once observed, strongly indicate that a woman is most likely pregnant, especially when coupled with any of the presumptive symptoms she may be experiencing. Probable signs of pregnancy include, but are not limited to:

- Hegar's sign—the softening of the uterine cervix and lower uterine segment (determined during a pelvic examination).
- Abdominal bloating or enlargement.
- Increased pigmentation of the skin around the woman's face, stomach, or surrounding the nipples on the breasts.
- Change in the size of the uterus (i.e., the uterus has an increased width and length, typically about five times the normal size).
- Uterine ballottement—when the lower uterine segment or cervix is tapped by a health care practitioner's fingers during a pelvic examination, the sensation of the fetus floating upward then sinking backward is felt.

- Striae gravidarum—the presence of dark streaking to the skin of the abdomen.
- Braxton Hicks contractions—painless uterine contractions beginning around week 12 and occurring throughout the pregnancy. These contractions typically cease with walking or other forms of exercise. Unlike uterine contractions associated with labor, Braxton Hicks do not cause the cervix to dilate.
- Positive pregnancy test. This can be misleading if the test is performed too early or too late following a missed period. For example, a positive pregnancy test could also be the result of an ectopic pregnancy or an abnormal growth of a fertilized egg (e.g., hydatiform mole).
- Palpating fetal parts. The health care practitioner may be able to palpate a woman's abdomen and feels parts of the fetus's body.

Definitive Signs

Definitive signs of pregnancy are those that directly confirm that a woman is pregnant. These include:

- Blood tests to confirm the presence, and quantity, of the pregnancy hormone HCG (human chorionic gonadotropin). These levels rise then predictably fall during the early weeks of pregnancy.
- Sonogram—a noninvasive diagnostic test that uses sound waves to explore the uterus to identify, and confirm, the presence of a fetus.
- Identifying a fetal heartbeat. A growing fetus has a unique heartbeat that can be detected using a stethoscope, fetoscope, or electronic device called a fetal doppler. The typical fetal heart rate is fast and ranges from 110 to 150 beats per minute compared to a woman's heart rate of 80 to 100 beats per minute.
- Fetal X-ray. Although not widely used in the United States or other industrialized nations, an X-ray can be used to determine and identify growing fetal bony structures present within the uterus.

23. Is teen pregnancy dangerous?

A pregnant teen is susceptible to unique medical risks for complications that could be dangerous to a teen mother or her baby. Although teen mothers can experience an uneventful pregnancy and delivery without complications, teen mothers are often at particular risk because of several factors like lack of, or insufficient, prenatal care, poor nutrition, smoking, or drug use. Research has suggested that a teenage girl's uterus is biologically immature, so there is an increased incidence of complications during pregnancy or at the time of delivery that can be further compounded by the multiple sociodemographic factors common among pregnant teens.

Teen mothers are at significant risk for developing high blood pressure during pregnancy (i.e., pregnancy-induced hypertension, or PIH). The exact mechanism for why this type of hypertension develops is unclear, but it frequently occurs in pregnant women at extremes of age (i.e., older pregnant women or younger teenage women). Although hypertension during pregnancy can often be controlled if it is monitored carefully and a woman has a balanced diet and sufficient exercise, teen mothers often lack the resources or ability to obtain regular prenatal care and often have a diet low in protein and fiber, high in sodium, and often consisting mostly of fast or processed foods. Hypertension in pregnancy can escalate to a more worrisome condition called preeclampsia. Preeclampsia is a worsening form of hypertension during pregnancy where the blood pressure remains persistently high, needed protein starts to leave the body and concentrate in the urine, and there is generalized swelling to the hands, feet, and face. The persistent high blood pressure can damage organs within the body, especially the liver and kidneys, or lead to the onset of seizures or a stroke. Like pregnancy-induced hypertension, the mechanism for why preeclampsia develops is also unclear; causes for its development include a systemic inflammatory response, metabolic abnormalities, or abnormalities in the development of the placenta. Medications can control the progression of preeclampsia, but, like hypertension, medications for blood pressure control often result in growth disruption in the baby.

Teen mothers are also at risk for premature birth. A full-term pregnancy ends at 39 or 40 weeks of gestation; teen mothers often give birth earlier. Babies born early are typically smaller and have a low birth weight (i.e., 3 to 5 pounds) or very low birth weight (less than 3 pounds). If a teen mother remains sexually active during pregnancy, the risk of contracting a sexually transmitted disease (STD) increases. Untreated STDs can lead to the development of preterm labor and possibly result in a premature birth. These small babies are at significant risk for a host of medical complications that can affect the baby's brain, lungs, digestive organs, or vision. These babies often require prolonged care in a neonatal intensive care unit (NICU) and, if complications develop, profound cognitive and developmental impairments can occur that are often permanent (e.g., cerebral palsy, blindness).

Teen mothers are also at high risk to develop depression during and after pregnancy. Many teen mothers cannot participate in school, lack financial resources for food or housing, and are overwhelmed by the prospect of impending motherhood. Although some teen mothers have support from family, friends, or the father of the baby, many face social isolation or being shunned within their communities that can lead to stress and worsen symptoms of existing depression or lead to the development of depression and anxiety. Limited medications for treating depression are approved for use in pregnancy, however, and mental health services are often unavailable, inconsistent, or inaccessible for teen parents.

24. What can I expect to happen in each trimester?

A typical pregnancy is approximately 40 weeks gestation in length but can range anywhere from 37 to 42 weeks gestation. It is divided into three trimesters: the first trimester is from conception through the end of week 12, the second trimester is weeks 13 through 26, and the third trimester is weeks 27 through delivery of the baby. Each trimester lasts about 12–13 weeks, or 3 months. Each trimester comes with its own specific hormonal and physiologic changes for both the mother and the baby. Being aware of the ways that the baby is growing and how her body changes can help a teen mother better prepare herself for these changes as they happen.

First Trimester

The first trimester begins with conception and lasts through the end of the 12th week of gestation. Conception usually occurs about or within 2 weeks after the last normal menstrual period. From conception onward, a woman's body goes through significant changes internally as it begins to accommodate the growing baby. In the first few weeks after conception, a woman's hormone levels change dramatically. The uterus begins to grow to support both the placenta and the fetus. A woman's blood supply begins to increase to help carry oxygen and nutrients to the growing fetus, and her heart rate begins to increase to be able to bring that increased blood supply consistently to the placenta and fetus.

Because of the rapid changes within her body, a woman may experience symptoms like fatigue, morning sickness, headaches, breast tenderness, or constipation. The next menstrual period is missed, signaling to a woman that she may be pregnant. Pregnancy is often confirmed in the first trimester.

The baby changes and grows rapidly during the first trimester. It will develop most of its organs by the end of the third month. The risk of miscarriage is highest during the first trimester, so it is imperative for a woman to avoid smoking, drugs, and alcohol, and to maintain a healthy diet with supplemental vitamins and folic acid as needed. Prenatal care begins in the first trimester and continues throughout the remainder of the pregnancy.

Second Trimester

The second trimester is weeks 13 through 26 of gestation. This is typically the most comfortable trimester for women: the uterus grows and rises out of the pelvis, relieving pressure off her bladder and decreasing her frequent urination. A woman recognizes a return of her energy level, she can sleep at night, and her early pregnancy symptoms are disappearing. The uterus continues to grow, and a woman will begin to look pregnant; loose, larger size, or maternity clothing will be needed. Weight gain, increased hunger, increased breast size, and Braxton Hicks contractions will occur. Exercise, healthy food choices, and continuing to avoid harmful substances are essential. Common physical complaints during the second trimester include backaches, leg cramps, heartburn, harmless vaginal discharge, and nasal discharge.

The baby continues to grow. The baby will be active within the uterus, turning and moving its arms and legs regularly. A woman will feel the frequent kicks or flutters regularly along with the times the baby is quiet. Important organs like the brain, heart, lungs, and kidneys can be visualized and monitored by ultrasound scans. The baby's sex can also be determined at this time. The baby's physical features are becoming defined and can be seen by high-resolution ultrasonography if available.

Third Trimester

The third trimester lasts from week 27 of gestation until the baby is born. The frequency of visits to the health care practitioner will occur more regularly and closer monitoring of blood pressure, the baby's heart rate, measuring the growth of the uterus, and checking for any signs of impending labor. The health care practitioner will check the baby's position in the uterus and assess for any changes to the cervix (e.g., shortening, dilatation) to determine if labor is imminent. A screening for Group B strep will occur at 35 to 37 weeks so, if positive, a woman can be given antibiotics when labor begins or when her water breaks.

The baby will begin to deposit more fat rapidly. Room inside the uterus is decreasing, and a woman will begin to be more uncomfortable as she approaches delivery. She will likely feel more pressure, fullness, and heaviness in her abdomen, lower back, and legs. Sleep is difficult and she will be more short of breath and become easily tired. Irregular contractions will occur, but some may be prolonged and painful. A woman should not travel far from where she is planning to deliver and should avoid prolonged car rides, long walks, or anything that could cause her to fall (e.g., snow, ice, or stairs).

25. Will I need any special prenatal care?

Prenatal care is the health care a woman receives while she is pregnant. Prenatal care should begin early in the pregnancy to provide the most benefit to the mother and her baby. It includes regular checkups and different kinds of specialized tests from a health care practitioner. The goal of prenatal care is to keep both the mother and baby healthy throughout the pregnancy. Prenatal care can also identify problems early on so treatment can be implemented or to prevent other problems from developing.

Teen mothers may have financial constraints, lack health insurance, or have cultural or language barriers that make them less likely to receive early and adequate prenatal care. They are more likely to smoke during pregnancy, be unmarried, have inadequate nutrition, and give birth to low birth weight or preterm babies. Teen mothers are also at high risk for developing high blood pressure and anemia during pregnancy. Because a teen mother has multiple physical, emotional, social, and environmental factors that can impact her pregnancy and the health of her baby, she requires specialized prenatal care to ensure all these influencing factors are addressed comprehensively.

Prenatal care for teen mothers initially focuses on the mother's physical health and well-being and the adequate growth and development of the baby. Along with a complete physical examination, a mother will be tested for sexually transmitted infections (STIs) and screened for them regularly at follow-up visits. Additional routine diagnostic tests like blood tests and ultrasound scans will also occur or be planned for at predictable intervals throughout the pregnancy during the follow-up visits. The mother will have her blood pressure closely watched, her weight gain monitored, the growth of the baby evaluated, and the fetal heart rate verified. Because there are known complications associated with teen pregnancy, rigorous screening for the development of these conditions will likely occur at each visit. Prenatal care visits will occur monthly during the early portion of the pregnancy but will increase in frequency as the pregnancy advances and happen weekly toward the time of delivery. Follow-up visits may also occur more often if complications develop or if a teen mother, or the baby, requires closer monitoring.

Important education and additional surveillance will also occur during the prenatal care visits for teen mothers. Mothers will receive ongoing education for healthy eating to ensure they are getting adequate folic acid, calcium, iron, and other essential nutrients. Activity and exercise will be monitored and assessed along with physical discomforts, mood, and energy level. Health care practitioners will be especially focused on monitoring a teen mother's environment and assessing her for the use of any drugs, alcohol or tobacco, risky behaviors, abuse from partners, peers, or parents, housing adequacy, and her exposure to any dangers or violence in the neighborhood or community. Health care practitioners have a network of resources, including social workers, to assist teen mothers when needed.

Prenatal care also establishes the schedule of childbirth classes a teen mother should attend to prepare her for labor and delivery of the baby. In addition, the health care practitioner will connect a teen mother with resources outside of childbirth classes to help build upon, and improve, a teen mother or teen parents' self-sufficiency and ability to transition to parenthood. Information about birth control is also provided to prevent future pregnancies. Parenting classes can benefit both teen parents and their families; these classes promote self-reliance while encouraging and supporting teens to complete high school or pursue advanced education or vocational training.

Prenatal care often occurs at a health care practitioner's office or within a health care facility. However, teens have unique circumstances that may prevent them from accessing prenatal care in traditional settings. Specialized prenatal care is now being offered in alternative settings like high schools, community centers, churches, in the home, at a discrete location, or in mobile units that bring care directly to mothers. Group prenatal care is gaining increasing popularity, especially with teen mothers and teen parents. In this model, small cohorts of mothers with similar gestational ages or due dates and needs are managed by one or two clinicians and sometimes a social worker. Designed to be efficient and cost effective, each mother is assessed and evaluated individually, but education is given

to the group. Current evidence suggests that participants in group prenatal care have better prenatal knowledge, feel better prepared for labor
and delivery, and are more likely to initiate and sustain breastfeeding after
delivery.

26. Are my baby and I covered under my parents' health insurance?

The landscape for insurance coverage in the United States changed dramatically under the Obama administration with the passage of the Affordable Care Act (ACA) in March 2010. Although many of the provisions
of the law were delayed until 2014, some parts of the law went into effect
immediately after the legislation was enacted. One of the most significant
provisions in the health care reform law that was implemented in 2010
was the extension of dependent coverage up to age 26 to assure that all
young adults had affordable health care coverage. Prior to the ACA, most
teens were no longer covered under their parent's health insurance by age
18 or only until the time they graduated from college.

Under the ACA, young adults, married or unmarried, can choose to
stay on their parent's insurance or enroll in an employer's health care plan
if they are working. However, spouses of young adults, or other dependents, are not covered under a parent's health insurance plan. However,
for pregnant teens on their parent's health insurance plan, coverage for
expenses related to the pregnancy, delivery, or follow-up care will only
occur if the individual insurance plan provides for maternity coverage. In
most situations, a teen covered under a parent's health insurance plan has
no coverage for the baby once it is born. There are few plans, if any, that
cover the dependents of dependents. Without proper planning, a baby is
born uninsured.

There are some options for a teen mother to explore to provide adequate health care insurance for the baby. A social worker can help navigate these options. State-funded health insurance (e.g., Medicaid) is
a common source of support for most infants; however, citizenship and
low-income requirements must be met for a child or family to qualify.
Each state has its own laws about eligibility for Medicaid. A baby born to
a mother enrolled in Medicaid or the Child Health Insurance Program
(CHIP) at the time of the birth is likely eligible for deemed newborn
coverage. This coverage begins at birth and lasts for one year, regardless of
any changes in the household income during that period. If one or both

parents are working and has health insurance through their employer, it may be possible to add the baby as a dependent to one insurance plan. However, insurance premiums can be costly and adding a dependent, regardless of their age or needs, can significantly increase those costs. At the present time, there is an opportunity to purchase health insurance for a baby called a "child-only" policy on the health care marketplace. Child-only health plans are insurance policies in which no parent or guardian is covered, and the policyholder is age 18 or younger. A grandparent, guardian, or other relative can pay for a child-only plan.

Most insurance plans, however, may require the baby to have a Social Security number prior to establishing a health insurance policy for the baby. Some group health insurance plans may allow a baby to be added as a dependent without a Social Security number. The easiest way to obtain a Social Security number for a baby is to complete a birth registration form at the time the baby is delivered. If the baby is not delivered in a hospital, or the birth registration form was not completed at the time of the birth, a parent can visit the local Social Security Administration office and request a number in person.

27. How will I know if I'm in labor?

Labor encompasses a variety of physical signs and symptoms that surround childbirth. The process of childbirth starts with contractions of the uterus and ends with the delivery of the baby. However, each woman's pregnancies are different, and each woman follows a different course, and experiences symptoms, individually. Although the onset of labor can be sudden, a woman's body goes through subtle changes throughout the pregnancy that prepare her for the ultimate delivery of the baby.

Uterine contractions can begin late in the first trimester but typically begin in some form in the second trimester and into the third trimester. Known as Braxton Hicks contractions, these uterine contractions are often brief and episodic. Braxton Hicks contractions are usually harmless but can sometimes be confused for uterine contractions associated with labor. Often brought on by dehydration or increased physical activity, Braxton Hicks contractions disappear with rest or position changes. Sometimes walking or stretching can also make them go away. During a Braxton Hicks contraction the baby is still active, and its movement can be felt by the mother. As the pregnancy progresses, the Braxton Hicks contractions become more noticeable. When noticed, the contractions have been described as a mildly uncomfortable tightening of the abdomen, slight pressure sensations felt across the abdomen, or like mild menstrual cramps. Also called "warm-up exercises" in preparation for labor, Braxton Hicks contractions are thought to help train the uterus for eventual labor and help the cervix start to efface, or thin out, closer to the time of delivery. Braxton Hicks contractions can last up to 30 seconds, happen irregularly anywhere from one to two times per hour or a few times per day.

Although Braxton Hicks contractions are harmless, a woman needs to be aware of the signs of premature labor to not confuse Braxton Hicks contractions for something more serious. Premature labor is the onset of labor prior to 37 weeks gestation. In premature labor, uterine contractions are noticeable; they are often felt as cramping pain in the lower abdomen that may be frequent or constant, low dull back pain that may be frequent or constant, or some combination of both. A woman may also feel increased pelvic pressure if the baby is descending or being pushed into the pelvis. Gastrointestinal cramps may also occur with or without diarrhea. An increase in vaginal discharge may be seen, or leaking of amniotic fluid may be noted. Bleeding is a true warning sign that requires immediate attention.

Since premature labor can be a common complication for teen mothers, she should lie on her left side with a pillow between her legs and contact her health care practitioner. She should describe her symptoms in as much detail as possible and follow the directions of the health care practitioner. Typically, an evaluation is necessary, often at the hospital or in a health care practitioner's office or clinic. An evaluation includes checking the baby and the uterus, often with ultrasound, and monitoring of the baby's heart rate and uterine contractions. Medications to stop uterine contractions and accelerate the baby's lung and brain maturity may be given. Admission to the hospital for prolonged monitoring or delivery of the baby may occur.

Most women can anticipate common physical signs that labor is impending or likely to begin soon. Labor is not a rapid process, and a woman's body goes through gradual changes leading up to the onset of active labor. About 2 to 4 weeks prior to the beginning of labor, most women will have a noticeable sensation that the baby "dropped," or lightening, as the baby begins to descend into the pelvis. She will likely have less shortness of breath but an increasing feeling of fullness in the pelvic area and an increased need to urinate frequently. As the baby continues to descend, lower back pain increases because the muscles and joints, especially in the hips and pelvis, begin to stretch and shift. The hormone relaxin loosens the ligaments all over a woman's body, especially before labor, making the joints feel looser, and lets the pelvis open to allow more room for the baby. Muscles begin to relax also, including the rectal muscles, so loose bowel movements, gas, or diarrhea are normal and common. Women should maintain their intake of fluids in the last few weeks leading up to the onset of labor.

Women may notice that their weight gain levels off or stops in the final weeks of pregnancy. The appetite decreases and women eat less. The baby, however, maintains or continues to gain weight. Women may observe fluctuating energy levels. Sleep becomes more difficult because of the physical discomforts, so napping is common and encouraged. Alternatively, women may also experience bursts of energy and an overwhelming desire to get the home ready for a new baby, which is known as "nesting." Women are advised to take advantage of opportunities to rest and to not overexert themselves doing tasks.

As the uterus prepares for delivery and the cervix begins to thin out and open, the mucus plug that blocks the cervix is often passed all at once or in pieces. Vaginal discharge increases and becomes thicker, pink, or red-tinged and without odor; this "bloody show" is a reliable indicator that the onset of labor is imminent. The uterus will continue to contract more regularly and begin its work to dilate the cervix and move the baby into the birth canal.

Uterine contractions differ from Braxton Hicks contractions; they get progressively stronger and do not ease up if a woman changes position. They increase in frequency and duration, becoming noticeably more painful and uncomfortable. The intensity of the contractions builds and can last for several day without changing. Uterine contractions are usually felt more across the abdomen, leaving the abdomen to feel firm or hard (like the forehead) for the duration of a contraction. During uterine contractions, a woman may break the bag of amniotic fluid spontaneously and see or feel a noticeable gush of fluid. A spontaneous break of the "bag of water" occurs in only 15% of women and can occur with or without uterine contractions.

A woman will see her health care practitioner weekly or more frequently in the final weeks of pregnancy. Her health care practitioner will teach her signs and symptoms to alert her that labor has started and when she should call the health care practitioner. The health care practitioner should always be called at any time if a woman notices any vaginal bleeding or bright red vaginal discharge or if her water breaks and the fluid is green, brown, or malodorous that would indicate the baby could be in trouble. Blurred vision, visual changes, increased swelling of the hands and feet, and severe headache or shortness of breath are other symptoms that should be reported immediately. As the uterine contractions progress, a woman typically notifies her health care practitioner when they are about 4 to 5 minutes apart for an hour and last about 30 to 70 seconds. The health care practitioner will determine if a woman needs to go to the hospital or if she can remain home to allow labor to progress.

28. What can I expect when it's time to deliver the baby?

Once labor begins the uterus starts to contract regularly to continue to open the cervix and push the baby further down into the birth canal. The main purpose of labor is to open the cervix wide enough (i.e., about 10 centimeters in diameter) to allow the baby's head and body to pass through while providing enough force to have the baby be delivered. Labor is a natural process, and each woman's labor is unique. Although most women follow a likely sequence of events from the beginning or onset of labor to the end, labor can be unpredictable, thus requiring skilled health care practitioners who know how to monitor the progress of labor and how well a mother and baby are tolerating the labor process. The labor process can be best understood by breaking it down into stages.

Stage I

The first stage of labor begins with the onset of regular uterine contractions that progressively increase to cause the cervix to dilate, or open, and shorten, or efface. This pattern of regular contractions allows the baby to descend and move into the birth canal. The first stage of labor is the longest of the three stages and is broken down into two phases: early or latent labor and active labor.

During early labor, the cervix begins to dilate and efface. Contractions will begin as mild but increase with notable frequency and intensity. Early labor varies in length or duration. For first-time mothers it can last hours or days; labor will often become shorter for subsequent pregnancies. Early labor is not particularly uncomfortable. During this phase, most women can remain at home and utilize activities like going for a walk, relaxation, breathing exercises, changes in position, back rubs, or taking a shower or bath for comfort.

Active labor begins after the cervix dilates to 6 centimeters and ends when the cervix dilates to 10 centimeters. During this phase uterine contractions are stronger, closer together, and last longer. Many women experience nausea or vomiting, as well as leg cramps and back pain or pressure. If the bag of water around the baby has not broken, it will likely rupture now, or the health care practitioner may opt to rupture it manually to make labor progress. Most women are very uncomfortable during this phase, but comfort techniques (e.g., focused breathing, pressure points) for natural childbirth can effectively manage pain. However, if those techniques are not successful, pain medication or regional pain relief like epidural or spinal anesthesia may be an option.

Active labor can last from 4 to 8 hours. A woman can expect that, on average, her cervix will dilate about 1 centimeter per hour. The health care practitioner, a labor coach, or a support person can assist a laboring woman to manage discomforts by employing the skills learned from childbirth preparation classes. Pain-relieving techniques include position changes, use of a birthing ball, a shower or tub bath, walking and stretching during contractions, or the use of massage on pressure points. Ice chips or sips of water, popsicles, or clear juices can help keep a woman hydrated throughout the labor process.

The last part of the active phase of labor, transition, can be particularly intense and painful. The uterine contractions are closer together and can last 60 to 90 seconds with increased pressure in the lower back and pelvis. The increased pressure creates an urge to push. However, the cervix might not be fully dilated, so the health care practitioner will feel the cervix and measure its dilatation manually by inserting one or two fingers into the vagina and gently palpating the cervix and the baby's head. Pushing may be discouraged if the cervix is not fully dilated. However, if the cervix is adequately dilated and the baby's head is in a good position within the birth canal, pushing with contractions can begin to deliver the baby.

Stage II

The second stage of labor begins when the cervix is completely dilated (i.e., 10 centimeters) and ends with the birth of the baby. Uterine contractions continue to push the baby down the birth canal. As the baby moves through the birth canal, a woman will feel increased or intense pressure, like an urge to have a bowel movement. This pressure helps a woman know when to push and bear down. The health care practitioner will instruct and coach a woman to push with each contraction. The contractions continue to be strong, but they may spread out a bit and give a woman some time to rest. The length of the second stage, however, is dependent on the size of the baby, the strength of the contractions, the mother's energy level and ability to push effectively, and if she has given birth before.

Delivery of the baby's head is controlled by the health care practitioner to gently guide it out of the birth canal and prevent injury to the vagina and the surrounding tissues. The baby's mouth and nose may be suctioned to help clear its airway in preparation for taking its first breath. Once the baby's shoulders pass under the pelvic bones, the infant can be firmly grasped by the health care practitioner to help guide the remainder of the baby's body out of the birth canal. The baby will be placed on the mother's abdomen, dried, and stimulated to cry. Once the umbilical cord stops pulsating, it will be clamped and cut. If the baby is transitioning well after delivery, it will be placed directly on the mother's chest to gradually warm up. Breastfeeding may be initiated while bonding continues.

Stage III

After the birth of the baby, the uterus continues to contract to push out the placenta (afterbirth). The placenta usually delivers about 5 to 15 minutes after the baby arrives. The placenta should deliver in one piece and is easily removed from the vagina. The placenta will be inspected by the health care provider to ensure that it detached off the uterine wall completely. If pieces or fragments are missing, the health care provider may gently explore the uterus to try to retrieve the lost pieces. Fragments of placental tissue left within the uterus prevent it from contracting fully and may lead to persistent bleeding.

Once the integrity of the placenta is confirmed, the health care practitioner will inspect the vagina and surrounding tissues for any injuries like lacerations or tears. If any repair is needed, the health care practitioner will use sutures to close any large open areas. Once the repairs are completed, the mother will be bathed, and ice will be applied to the vaginal area for comfort and control of any swelling. The mother will be encouraged to eat and drink fluids and to pass urine when ready.

Stage IV

The final stage is the recovery phase. Women are often tired or fatigued following the birth process but also may feel elation, relief, or excitement. Breastfeeding should continue to promote contraction of the uterus and bonding with the baby. New mothers are encouraged to continue to eat and drink and to walk around when they feel ready. New mothers use the bathroom to pass urine frequently and will be able to shower. The baby will be monitored and assessed at regular intervals and, when both the mother and infant are stable, will be sent home.

29. Can I have a normal birth, or do I have to have a cesarean birth?

Babies can enter the world in only one of two ways. A pregnant woman can have a vaginal birth or a surgical, cesarean birth. Regardless of the method of delivery, the goal for both is the safe delivery of a healthy baby. A vaginal delivery is the normal, preferred route of delivery for a baby. Women who undergo vaginal birth avoid having major abdominal surgery and its associated risks like severe bleeding, scarring, infections, and prolonged pain or discomfort and anesthesia reactions. After a vaginal birth, hospital stays are often shorter and recovery time is faster compared to a cesarean birth. Vaginal birth also permits breastfeeding and bonding with the baby to be initiated sooner.

The baby also benefits from a vaginal birth. During a vaginal delivery, the muscles involved in the birth process work to gently squeeze out fluid from the baby's lungs and help prevent respiratory complications at birth. Babies are also exposed to healthy microorganisms within the birth canal that are believed to support a baby's immune system and protect and colonize its intestinal tract.

Despite the many benefits of a vaginal birth, there are also some risks associated with it. During a vaginal delivery, it is not uncommon for the skin or tissues around the vagina to stretch or tear while the baby is moving through the birth canal. Sometimes the stretching and tearing can be severe enough to require repair with sutures. In addition, there could be injury to the pelvic muscles, making them weaker and causing a woman to have issues controlling her bowel functions or urine like leaking or dribbling urine with laughing, coughing, or sneezing. Women may also experience prolonged pain or swelling to the vaginal area or to the skin of the perineum.

A cesarean birth is the delivery of a baby through a surgical incision through a woman's lower abdomen and uterus. Although cesarean births are common procedures, they are complicated and carry significant risks for the mother and baby. Cesarean deliveries are often reserved for emergent situations or for specific medical conditions.

Emergency situations are often the most common indication for a woman to undergo a cesarean birth. Despite the normal progress of labor, the baby may not be able to tolerate the stress of repeated, prolonged uterine contractions. Babies who experience fetal distress will have sudden or prolonged drops, or decelerations, in their heart rate, signifying compromised circulation within the baby. Repeated, prolonged episodes of fetal distress can cause permanent brain injury to a baby. Similarly, during labor there is a risk that the umbilical cord can slip down into the birth canal and get trapped or squeezed during contractions or by the baby's head. This cord prolapse cuts off circulation to the baby and results in rapid, sustained fetal distress, thus emergent surgical delivery is necessary. The placenta can also be a source of concern; women, especially teen mothers with high blood pressure or preeclampsia, are susceptible to the placenta suddenly dislodging from the uterine wall. Known as placental abruption, this immediately deprives the baby of any oxygen or circulation, can cause severe bleeding for the mother, and is another cause for emergent surgical delivery.

There are medical conditions that, once identified, can allow a cesarean delivery to be planned or scheduled. Teen mothers, due to their immature body stature, may have a pelvis that is too small or narrow to accommodate a full-term baby. If the baby is believed to have a head or body too large for a woman to safely deliver vaginally, a cesarean birth is the safest delivery route for the mother and baby. Similarly, teen mothers are also more likely to have high blood pressure or gestational diabetes, which can also make a baby too small and too fragile to be delivered vaginally, so the option of a cesarean delivery may be preferred. Babies are expected to remain in the uterus and enter the birth canal head down, especially toward the end of the pregnancy. However, some babies may lie sideways or have their feet, buttocks, or face be the presenting body part. Known as a breech baby, this malposition can be dangerous for a baby, so a vaginal delivery is avoided.

With the improvements and advances in prenatal care and the use of sophisticated ultrasonography, it is possible for health care practitioners to identify and diagnose congenital defects in a baby during pregnancy. These defects, like congenital cardiac abnormalities or hydrocephalus, can often put a baby at risk for injury both during labor and throughout the delivery process. Babies with identified anomalies or defects are often safer to be delivered by cesarean birth.

Active genital infections would also increase the likelihood for a woman to require a cesarean birth. Infections like active herpes lesions or HIV disease exposes the baby to potentially harmful microorganisms that could create health issues for the baby. To prevent the baby from meeting any vaginal tissues or membranes that contain harmful microorganisms, a cesarean birth is recommended.

The mother's overall health can also determine her need for a cesarean birth. Mothers with chronic cardiac, respiratory, neurologic, or musculoskeletal conditions may not be able to physically tolerate the demands of labor or be able to push at the time of delivery. In addition, mothers who develop complications during pregnancy like gestational diabetes or pre-eclampsia may also not be able to tolerate labor if their condition worsens or the baby becomes at risk by prolonged labor or the delivery process.

30. Am I at risk for any complications because I'm a teenager?

Any woman going through labor and the birth process is susceptible to any of the common complications associated with childbirth. Teen mothers, as a unique population, are at no greater risk for these complications occurring compared to other women. Although teen mothers are more susceptible to medical complications developing during pregnancy (e.g., gestational hypertension, preeclampsia, or gestational diabetes), teen mothers typically have less incidence of complications during labor and delivery. One complication most seen in teen mothers is a condition called cephalopelvic disproportion (CPD). CPD occurs when the infant's head or its body is too large to fit through the mother's pelvis and into the birth canal. Teen mothers who have not completed their natural bodily growth process may have a pelvis that is too small or too narrow for a baby to safely pass into the birth canal. For most cases of true CPD in teen mothers, a cesarean birth is the safest method of delivery.

The complications of childbirth can be nonemergent or emergent. Although health care practitioners attempt to identify any risk factors for complications and remain vigilant for their onset, there is no way to accurately predict if or when complications will occur during the childbirth process.

Nonemergent complications are those that occur but do not pose an immediate threat to the mother or her baby, so emergency interventions are not needed. The most common nonemergent complication is the failure of labor to progress. Sometimes uterine contractions weaken, or the regularity or frequency of the uterine contractions becomes disorganized or sporadic. When labor fails to progress, the cervix does not dilate enough or in a timely manner, so the baby does not effectively descend into the birth canal. If labor is not progressing, the health care practitioner may give a mother additional medication to increase the contractions or to speed up labor. If these interventions fail, a cesarean birth may be necessary.

Another possible nonemergent complication is a mother's water, or bag of water, breaking too early. Labor typically begins within 24 hours of a mother's water breaking; if labor does not begin and the pregnancy is at or near term, a health care practitioner may induce labor. However, if a pregnant mother's water breaks before 34 weeks of pregnancy, she will likely be monitored in the hospital. Infection can become a major concern if a mother's water breaks early and labor does not commence on its own.

Another common nonemergent complication is tears or lacerations to the skin and tissues surrounding the vagina during the delivery process. The pressure of the baby's head passing through the birth canal can overstretch the tissues to the point they tear to allow the delivery to happen. Some health care practitioners may see the tissues becoming jeopardized and may opt to perform an episiotomy to prevent any jagged or irregular tears to the vaginal tissues. If a tear occurs, it may be small enough to heal on its own. More serious tears, or an episiotomy itself, requires stitches to repair the injury and promote proper healing.

Emergency complications are a real possibility during childbirth for any mother. Health care practitioners are particularly vigilant for the early identification of these complications so emergency interventions can be implemented. A common complication that may require emergency intervention is abnormal changes in the baby's heart rate. During childbirth, the baby's heart rate fluctuates; however, it can suddenly drop or accelerate out of normal range, signifying a problem. Health care practitioners will try noninvasive maneuvers like position changes or giving the mother oxygen to correct the baby's heart rate and improve blood flow to the baby. If the abnormal heart rate persists, emergency delivery may be indicated.

The baby's umbilical cord floats within the amniotic fluid during pregnancy. However, after a mother's water breaks, there is less fluid in the uterus, so the length of cord is in close contact with the baby's body and the uterine wall. The umbilical cord may get caught around the baby's arm or leg or become trapped between the baby's head and the cervix. In an extreme case the umbilical cord may slip down and drop out of the cervix in the vagina. Since the umbilical cord is attached to the placenta and the main lifeline for the baby, any compression or prolapse of the umbilical cord will compromise the baby's heart rate and circulation. If the baby does not receive enough oxygen, a condition called perinatal asphyxia can occur that, if persistent, can cause brain damage in the baby. When this situation occurs, emergency interventions or delivery is needed.

The placenta is a vital organ that serves as the baby's source of nutrients and oxygen during pregnancy. During labor, as uterine contractions become more frequent and intense, there is a possibility of the placenta suddenly separating completely from the uterine wall. Known as placental abruption, this emergency signifies the baby is deprived of oxygen and an emergent cesarean delivery must occur.

In most cases a baby progresses down the birth canal without problems. However, as the baby's head is born through the vagina, the baby's shoulders may get stuck underneath the pelvic bones (i.e., shoulder dystocia), preventing the completion of the delivery. Once discovered, the health care practitioner and the delivery team act quickly to employ a series of maneuvers to relieve the impingement and quickly complete the delivery. If unrelieved, an emergency cesarean delivery may be necessary.

The uterus can tear at any time during the childbirth process or not contract completely after the delivery of the baby and the placenta. Heavy bleeding, or hemorrhage, can follow. Health care practitioners have a variety of medications, interventions, or blood transfusions to employ to help minimize the bleeding and its effect on the mother. Maternal hemorrhage during the childbirth process has been identified as the most common cause of death for women worldwide.

31. Is my baby at risk for any medical complications because I'm a teenager?

Pregnant teen mothers are at risk for specific medical conditions that can also cause significant medical complications for their baby. Pregnant teens are more likely to be from a lower socioeconomic class that makes housing and access to adequate nutrition difficult. In place of healthy foods, teen mothers often consume highly processed or fast foods that are affordable or accessible. Because many teen mothers live at or below the poverty level, they are less likely to access adequate medical care for themselves or to seek regular prenatal care for their baby. The stress of insufficient resources for food, housing, or day-to-day needs also contributes to the increased incidence of pregnant teen mothers to engage in risky behaviors like smoking, alcohol, or drug use, or be exposed to violence. Further, teen mothers who remain sexually active during pregnancy and maintain unsafe sex practices, or have multiple partners, are at high risk for contracting harmful sexually transmitted infections (STIs).

Teen mothers also possess physiologic immaturity; their bodies and organ systems have not achieved their full functional or developmental status. Therefore, teen mothers are less likely to be able to manage the physical demands of pregnancy. Teen mothers are more likely to have anemia, a condition worsened by poor nutrition and a lack of proper monitoring and follow-up common with prenatal care. Pregnant teen mothers are also more likely to develop gestational diabetes, have high blood pressure, or develop preeclampsia.

The social and physiologic risks that may surround a pregnant teen mother impact the health and well-being of their baby. Pregnant teen mothers are more likely to experience premature birth and deliver a baby that is susceptible to a host of medical complications because of its small size, underdeveloped organs (especially the lungs), and lack of sufficient body weight. Pregnant teen mothers are also likely to deliver a low birth weight baby who weighs less than 5½ pounds (or less than 2,500 grams) that will delay the baby's full growth and development. If a pregnant teen has untreated STIs, the harmful microorganisms can cause pneumonia and respiratory issues for the newborn. Further, an untreated STI like syphilis can cause permanent blindness in a baby. Teen mothers who are HIV-positive may transmit the virus to their baby. The multiple complications a newborn may experience can ultimately lead to the baby's death in the immediate newborn period or within the first year of life.

Research also supports that infants born to teen mothers may also be at risk for social and cognitive issues. Infants of teen mothers may grow up with cognitive impairments that lead to lower academic achievement, repeating grades, poor performance on standardized tests, or profound learning disabilities. These children are also more likely to be involved in accidents during their childhood and early teen years. If the cycle of poverty continues, these children are more likely to be exposed to, or involved in, violence or enter the prison system. The likelihood of these children becoming teen parents themselves also increases.

32. What medical care does the baby need after it's born?

The baby's medical care begins while the mother is still pregnant. Prenatal care not only monitors the health status of the mother but also checks that the baby is growing properly. Tests like laboratory blood work or ultrasound identify any conditions or defects in the baby to allow early intervention if possible or to create a management and treatment plan for the time of delivery.

Immediately after birth the delivery team works to rapidly assess the baby and provide any support a baby may need in the first minutes of life. The baby will be quickly dried and stimulated to cry. A member of the delivery team will assign an Apgar score at 1 and 5 minutes of life. The Apgar score rates the baby's heart rate, muscle tone, and other signs to determine if the baby needs additional support (e.g., oxygen) or emergency care; a score of 7 to 10 is an ideal Apgar score. Once the baby is stabilized, it is kept warm either on the mother's chest by skin-to-skin contact or wrapped in baby blankets. Babies are encouraged to initiate breastfeeding immediately after birth. Vitamin K is given as an injection to promote blood clotting and prevent bleeding. Antibiotic ointment is placed in the baby's eyes to prevent any harmful microorganisms from the birth canal causing damage to the baby's eyes or vision.

During the first days of life, the baby is regularly assessed in the nursery by the health care team. Weight, length, and head circumference measurements are recorded. The number and character of the baby's bowel movements and the amount of urine passed are monitored. Feeding patterns and the amount taken at each feeding are closely monitored. The baby will have a full physical examination each day in the nursery by a health care practitioner to ensure the baby is adjusting well to extrauterine life.

Various screening tests occur during the immediate newborn period. Blood glucose levels may be monitored to ensure babies are being adequately fed to meet their metabolic needs. Bilirubin, a pigment formed in the baby's liver by the breakdown of hemoglobin and excreted in the bile, may be tested if the baby shows signs of jaundice or yellowing of the skin. Most states require a newborn screening test, which is a simple blood test from a heel stick that looks to identify conditions that can affect a child's long-term health or survival. These conditions include genetic, endocrine, and metabolic disorders that are not apparent at birth like phenylketonuria (PKU), cystic fibrosis, or sickle cell disease. This newborn screening is performed regardless of insurance coverage and in some states may be repeated in 1 to 2 weeks after birth.

Babies will require regular follow-up from a pediatrician during their first year of life. Babies are typically reevaluated by a pediatrician or other health care practitioner within 5 to 7 days after discharge from the hospital. At each follow-up visit the baby's weight, length, and head circumference will be checked. A full physical examination will be done to assess the baby's growth and development along with any achievement of developmental milestones. During these visits, the health care practitioner will review how the baby is doing and inform the mother or parents about what to expect next related to growth and development. A significant amount of teaching is provided to parents or families, and additional educational material is often provided. One of the most important aspects of these follow-up visits is the timely administration of vaccines.

Babies receive their first vaccine, hepatitis B, during the first days of life while in the nursery. Throughout the first year of life a baby requires vaccines to protect against diseases like rotovirus; influenza B; polio; pneumococcal pneumonia; diphtheria, tetanus, and pertussis (i.e., D-tap for children); measles, mumps, and rubella (MMR); and varicella (chickenpox). The schedule for these vaccines may vary, but typically babies receive them at 2, 4, and 6 months of life, and then at their first birthday. How these vaccines are administered (i.e., what is due may be given all at once or split into different times) is determined by the health care practitioner and the parent.

Aside from the routine checkups and vaccinations, babies can also experience sudden illnesses that may require an evaluation from a health care practitioner. A baby should be taken to a health care practitioner's office or clinic if the situation is not emergent. Examples of nonemergent signs include if the baby refuses to eat for several feedings in a row; has repeated episodes of vomiting or diarrhea; has a cold that does not improve or worsens; a rash; signs of dehydration like few wet diapers, no tears, or sunken eyes; and ear drainage or cannot stop crying. However, a baby should be taken to an emergency room if it has difficulty breathing; a seizure; is limp, unarousable, or sleeping more than usual; has any bleeding; an injury or poisoning; yellow skin or eyes; or a rectal temperature equal to or greater than 100.4 degrees Fahrenheit.

33. Will I be able to breastfeed?

Breast milk is considered the most ideal source of nutrition for infants. Mothers are encouraged to exclusively breastfeed their babies; this means the baby receives only breast milk and no additional forms of commercial infant formula until solid foods are introduced. The World Health Organization (WHO) recommends that mothers exclusively breastfeed their babies for the first 6 months of life and then continue breastfeeding combined with solid food for two years or for as long as the mother and baby desire. Some babies, however, may decrease the number of breastfeeds as they begin to be able to digest solid food.

The benefits of breastfeeding for both the baby and the mother have been supported by research. Breast milk helps protect the baby against allergies and other skin conditions. Because the proteins in breast milk are easier for the baby to digest, breastfed babies have less stomach upset, diarrhea, or constipation. The immunity-boosting antibodies in breast milk also prevent babies from developing ear infections, upper respiratory infections, urinary tract infections, inflammatory bowel disease, gastro-enteritis, and other viral infections common in children. Breastfed infants have a lower incidence of sudden infant death syndrome (SIDS), child-hood cancers, and childhood obesity.

Breastfeeding also benefits the mother. Mothers who breastfeed recover quicker from childbirth. Hormones released during lactation help keep the uterus contracted and lessens bleeding after delivery. Breastfeeding also reduces a woman's risk of breast and ovarian cancers developing later in life, along with lower incidence of high blood pressure, high choles-terol, rheumatoid arthritis, diabetes, and cardiovascular diseases. The higher levels of the hormone prolactin required for lactation also help suppress the hormones that cause ovulation, providing mothers with addi-tional protection against future pregnancies. Breastfeeding promotes the emotional and physician attachment between a mother and her baby. Breastfeeding is also economical and requires no special equipment. Therefore, any mother, regardless of age, can breastfeed as soon as breast development during puberty commences.

Breast development, including the necessary structures within the breast to produce and transport breast milk, begins for girls during puberty. There-fore, teen mothers are equipped to fully breastfeed their babies adequately and should be encouraged to do so after the baby is born. Lactation, or the secretion of milk from the mammary glands, is regulated by a feedback loop of hormones that begins during pregnancy. Breast size does not impact the ability to breastfeed; large and small-breasted women undergo the same pro-cesses to produce breast milk and have an equal milk supply.

The mammary glands are lobes or masses of tissue within the breast. Each lobe has a rich blood supply made up of a network of blood vessels and lactiferous ducts to transport milk. From birth until puberty there are only a few ducts present. Once puberty begins, the increased levels of the hormone estrogen causes the ducts to grow and enlarge. With each menstrual cycle the breast tissues respond to the repeated surges of estro-gen and progesterone. Women often complain of increased breast ten-derness, swelling of the breasts and irregular, temporary changes in breast size, breast heaviness, soreness, or pain for several days during a monthly menstrual cycle due to the hormonal influences.

During pregnancy, the increase in estrogen and progesterone causes the breast tissue to grow and enlarge. The breasts may remain tender and sensitive to touch throughout pregnancy. The nipples and the skin around them (i.e., the areolas) may become darker and expand. Small bumps on the surface of the areolas called Montgomery tubercles become more raised and prominent. The veins or blood vessels along the breasts become more visible and noticeable. The breasts may leak a thick, yellowish substance called colostrum beginning during the second trimester and continuing until after delivery.

Until the time of delivery, the amount of progesterone remains slightly higher than the amount of estrogen. Higher levels of progesterone support the development of breast tissue and its network of ducts but does not promote the secretion of breast milk. However, after delivery of the placenta the levels of progesterone drop dramatically, and the breast tissue becomes exposed to higher levels of the hormone prolactin. The breasts begin to produce large amounts of colostrum, which provides the baby with proteins and fat-soluble vitamins.

Breast milk begins to form within 24 to 48 hours after delivery due to the influence of prolactin. Prolactin production is stimulated by the baby suckling at the breast. Suckling stimulates receptors in the nipple to promote the secretion of prolactin. Suckling at one breastfeeding promotes prolactin release which, in turn, causes production and accumulation of breast milk for the next feeding.

The baby suckling at the breast (or the expression of milk using a mechanical breast pump) allows the breast milk to flow to the baby. Babies do not suck milk out of the breast; milk is ejected by the let-down reflex. This reflex causes the cells surrounding the breast tissues and ducts to contract to squeeze milk out. Although suckling is the major source of stimulation for the let-down reflex, some women's let-down reflex can be stimulated by the sight of their baby or by hearing it cry. In contrast, pain or alcohol can inhibit the let-down reflex.

The key to successful maintenance of breast milk production is sufficient suckling (or pumping) stimulation at each breastfeeding to maintain adequate secretion of prolactin and to remove accumulated milk from the milk ducts. If suckling stops, milk production ceases gradually.

34. How do I prevent getting pregnant again?

After giving birth, current recommendations by the American College of Obstetricians and Gynecologists (ACOG) advise women to wait at least 6 months or more after delivery before getting pregnant again. However, it is possible for women to get pregnant immediately after giving birth if they are sexually active. Most women are advised to avoid sexual intercourse for 4 to 6 weeks following delivery to allow proper healing of the vagina (or of a cesarean birth surgical incision) and prevent any infections in the uterus. Each woman, however, is unique; some may resume ovulation with or without a menstrual period within a month after delivery while other women take longer. Because fertility is unpredictable, the only way to prevent pregnancy from happening again, both immediately after delivery and long term, is for women to use some form of contraception.

The decision of which birth control method to use, and when to use it, following the birth of a baby depends on a few factors. First, if a woman plans to breastfeed her baby, her choices of birth control will be narrowed because several forms of hormonal contraception can interfere with lactation. Regardless of what method a woman chooses, it is important that she discuss her plans for birth control with her health care provider prior to delivery.

Barrier methods are the most popular form of birth control following delivery of a baby. Condoms, for example, are affordable, convenient, and effective at preventing pregnancy when used properly and consistently. A woman or couple can keep an ample supply of condoms on hand for resuming sexual activity. Diaphragms are another barrier method option. However, if a woman wants to use a diaphragm, she will need an examination by her health care practitioner postdelivery to check the fit and size of the diaphragm before it is used following delivery of a baby; childbirth changes the tone and shape of the vagina, so a specific type or size of diaphragm may be necessary. Because diaphragms require additional spermicidal lubricant and care to prevent the diaphragm from ripping or breaking down, they are not a popular option among teens.

If a woman is considering hormonal contraception, she will typically need to wait about 4 weeks following delivery. After childbirth, levels of estrogen in a woman's bloodstream are high; adding estrogen from various forms of birth control such as oral contraceptive pills (OCPs), hormonal patches, or vaginal rings could put a woman at risk for blood clots or other dangerous side effects. Estrogen levels begin to decline by approximately 4 weeks following delivery of a baby, so it is safer to initiate either combined hormonal OCPs, the hormonal patch, or the vaginal ring a month or more following delivery. If a woman is breastfeeding, estrogen-containing forms of birth control are avoided until breast milk production and supply are well established; estrogen may reduce the quantity and quality of breast milk. However, if a woman is breastfeeding, she may opt to use the "mini pill," or a progestin-only form of OCP. Although the mini pill is a good alternative for breastfeeding women, the mini pill requires a steady dose of hormone to be present in a woman's bloodstream; the mini pill must be taken at the same time each day as prescribed, without missing a dose, or its contraceptive effect is diminished.

Long-acting hormonal contraception can be initiated at the time of delivery of a baby or immediately thereafter. A woman can receive her first injection of Depo-Provera, a progestin-only form of birth control, immediately after giving birth or prior to discharge from the hospital without interfering with her ability to breastfeed. In addition, Depo-Provera taken immediately after delivery provides a woman 12 weeks of consistent birth control, allowing her to explore, and initiate, other birth control options by the time of her first postdelivery, follow-up appointment with her health care practitioner, or approximately 6 weeks after delivery. Intrauterine devices, or IUDs, were previously not considered for teenage girls. However, in recent years IUDs have become a popular birth long-acting hormonal birth control method because they last for five to ten years depending on the brand or type used, provide a consistent, reliable form of birth control, and have minimal side effects. However, IUDs do not prevent or protect a teenage girl from sexually transmitted infections (STIs). Some practitioners will insert an IUD immediately following delivery of a baby and the placenta because there is optimal visualization of the cervix to allow accurate placement of the IUD. Most health care practitioners will opt to insert an IUD from 4 to 6 weeks following delivery to minimize the risk of improper placement or infection.

Permanent sterilization procedures are often not an option for teenage mothers. Sterilization procedures are meant to be permanent and would eliminate the possibility of teenage girls having a baby in future years. These types of procedures (e.g., tubal ligation) are reserved for women who are finished having children.

35. Does having a baby in my teens affect my ability to have children in the future?

Fertility refers to a woman's ability to conceive a child or her ability to become pregnant. Having a baby as a teenager should have no impact on a woman's ability to have more children. However, there are certain medical conditions that could develop over time that could impair a woman's fertility regardless of when she may have given birth in the past.

Genetics play a major role in future fertility. If a woman has relatives (e.g., her mother or sisters) who struggled with fertility, her chances or experiencing similar issues is increased. Just because a woman had a baby in the past does not mean she will not experience issues with, or periods of, infertility in the future. Gynecologic and medical reasons, however, are primary causes for most women's fertility issues.

The ovaries are responsible for the production of the hormone estrogen that is necessary for an egg to be released during ovulation. Anything that interferes with the ovaries secreting their hormone or releasing an egg will result in a woman experiencing infertility. Conditions like polycystic ovarian syndrome (PCOS), hyperprolactinemia, or thyroid disorders can interrupt the normal hormonal feedback loop within a woman's body and prevent ovulation. Other medical conditions that may develop over time like poorly controlled diabetes, celiac disease, autoimmune disorders, cancers (especially those treated with radiation and chemotherapy), and ovarian surgeries can also interrupt the ovary's ability to function.

Structural or anatomic defects or injuries can also impede a woman's ability to conceive. Uterine or cervical abnormalities like polyps or fibroids can prevent sperm from entering the cervix or prevent the uterus from developing a consistent inner lining (i.e., endometrium) to allow a fertilized egg to implant. The fallopian tubes, which carry an egg to the uterus to be fertilized, can become scarred or damaged from untreated sexually transmitted infections (STIs), pelvic inflammatory disease (PID), or from surgery for an ectopic pregnancy thus preventing conception. Women who develop endometriosis may have lesions of endometrial tissue that surround or occlude the fallopian tubes or the uterus that would prevent successful conception. Women who have had lower abdominal or pelvic surgery, or had infections in those areas, can develop scar tissue that can adhere to the uterus, fallopian tubes, or ovaries and further impede a woman's ability to conceive. Obesity distorts a woman's hormonal feedback loop and further prevents regular ovulation.

Social and environmental factors can also cause infertility in women. Safe sex practices with intercourse and regular sexually transmitted infections (STIs) screenings for women with different sex partners or repeated episodes of unprotected intercourse help minimize the harmful damage from STIs. Smoking has been demonstrated to age the ovaries faster, cause premature depletion of a woman's inborn supply of eggs within the ovaries, and to cause chronic ovarian damage. Like smoking, excessive alcohol and drug use can also cause chronic, and permanent, damage to the ovaries. Environmental toxins like pollutants or contaminants in the air or drinking water and lead have been implicated as causes of women's infertility and for the development of birth defects if pregnancy should occur.

Recent research has demonstrated that shift work, especially night shift or shifts that begin during early morning hours, interrupt a woman's normal sleep cycle and her normal feedback loop of hormonal regulation. This disruption significantly impacts estrogen release and can be a cause of infertility. Caffeine, whether it is used to sustain shift work or as a drink of choice, has also been demonstrated to contribute to infertility when intake exceeds 200 mg/day or more than one or two 6- or 8-ounce cups per day. Sedentary lifestyles and lack of exercise or dieting with rapid weight loss alters a woman's secretion of progesterone and can also distort ovulation.

36. Are there any mental or emotional concerns I need to worry about during pregnancy or after giving birth?

Women, regardless of age, experience a wide range of emotions throughout their pregnancies and after delivery. However, research has demonstrated that teen mothers are more susceptible to most of the negative mental and emotional concerns during and after pregnancy compared to adult women. Although each teen mother is different, as a group or population teen mothers often are from low-income families or unstable home environments with limited financial resources. Teen mothers also have a higher incidence of experiencing pregnancy complications and have a minimal social network of family or friends because of their pregnancy. Teen mothers also experience more abuse or are likely to be in more abusive situations or relationships compared to adult women.

Because teen mothers have physical, social, and financial issues that surround their pregnancy, stress is a commonly reported complaint from teen mothers. Although each person manages stress differently, teen mothers, and teen parents, report more feelings of hopelessness, being powerless, and feeling overwhelmed from stress. Teens have few opportunities to test and develop effective coping strategies for managing stress. Persistent stress leads to sleeplessness, additional physical discomforts (e.g., tension, muscle soreness, headaches), and additional anxiety.

Anxiety can range from simple worries to panic attacks. Teen mothers reported increased anxiety about their health, the health of their baby, and the future. Teen mothers also reported persistent thoughts or concerns about being able to finish school or get a job, support, and keep their baby, maintain a relationship with the baby's father and his family, or be accepted by their own. Like stress, teen mothers have few opportunities to test and develop adequate coping skills to manage anxiety. Persistent anxiety and worry lead to additional stress and feelings of fear.

Teen mothers report feeling fearful about, or afraid of, the future. They are frightened about being pregnant, the changes their bodies go through, the complications that may develop, and the pain and uncertainty of labor and the childbirth process. Teen mothers also fear not having a "normal" baby and their abilities to be a successful parent with limited resources. Teen mothers also fear losing their circle of friends, their relationship with the baby's father, or being stigmatized or ostracized by their extended family, community, or religious group.

Following delivery of the baby, teen mothers are susceptible to the same emotional issues as adult women. Indeed, emotional issues are common after delivery, believed to be caused by the physical stress of the childbirth process and the sudden, dramatic physiologic and hormonal changes that occur within a woman's body following delivery of the baby and the placenta. The "Baby Blues" are common among women after delivery. Occurring within 1 to 2 weeks after birth, women report mood swings, periods of unexplained sadness, anxiety or feeling overwhelmed, difficulty concentrating, eating, or being able to care for themselves or their baby. Although these symptoms are often self-limiting, they can persist and develop into postpartum depression (PPD). PPD is a pervasive, ongoing condition that is real and can last indefinitely. Mothers experiencing PPD have varying emotions from sadness to dread. PPD can be debilitating; it is accompanied by feelings of extreme fatigue, worthlessness, panic attacks, and thoughts of harming themselves or their baby. Suicide, or harming the baby, is not uncommon in women who have untreated, or poorly treated, PPD. Fortunately, effective treatment options exist for PPD and the possible post-traumatic stress disorder (PTSD) that may develop following childbirth or after delivery. Parents or a strong social network of supportive people, in addition to proper treatment, can greatly impact a teen mother's positive recovery if diagnosed with any form of mental or emotional issues.

Because mental and emotional health issues are so common among teen mothers, rigorous screening processes are in place to help identify mothers at risk and expedite interventions. All women who have given birth, especially teen mothers, are carefully screened for the onset, or potential onset, of PPD using a reliable and valid screening tool within the first days after delivery and then at follow-up visits with a health care practitioner. In addition, pediatricians or other health care practitioners caring for a baby or child are acutely aware to assess the mother and her connection to, and interaction with the baby and her overall appearance, health, and coping to meet the needs of her baby or child. Health care practitioners will intervene immediately if they suspect, or confirm, that a teen mother may be experiencing any of the symptoms of PPD, PTSD, or any other mental or emotional issue. Social workers are an invaluable resource for any mother who requires intervention, referral, or follow-up.

Legal Concerns

37. Do I have to tell my parents I'm pregnant?

Any woman, including a teen mother, is not under any obligation to disclose whether she is pregnant to her parents or other family members. Some teen mothers may need to share the news about their pregnancy if they lack individual health insurance and are planning to use a parent's insurance coverage for their medical care and treatment. However, other options for insurance coverage are available for teen mothers if coverage under a parent's health insurance plan is nonexistent, insufficient, or withheld for any reason.

Research supports that teen mothers who have parental support during the pregnancy avoid many of the emotional, social, and financial complications common with teen pregnancy. Following delivery, parental support provides a smoother transition to parenthood for a teen mother. Therefore, sharing the truth about being pregnant could be beneficial for both a teen mother and her baby. However, not every family may be receptive or accepting of the news about a teen's pregnancy. Choosing a time to share the news about pregnancy may require planning and careful consideration.

First, a teen mother needs to evaluate her safety and if sharing the news about being pregnant would put her in jeopardy. If a teen mother feels she may be at risk for injury or violence she should choose to share her news in a safe location like a public place or have a trusted adult friend, social worker, or counselor accompany her. Having the father of the baby with her could be effective but may also worsen the situation depending on the nature of the couple's relationship or the relationship between the father of the baby and her family. It is recommended that significant family events like religious holidays or celebrations, birthdays, anniversaries, funerals, or family parties and gatherings be avoided as places or times to share news about a pregnancy. A teen mother disclosing her pregnancy status should expect the unexpected but realize, and accept, that she is the priority and focus and that she possesses the inner strength to be resilient and survive whatever consequence comes from telling her parents or family.

A teen mother needs to assess her own response and reaction to knowing she is pregnant. She should accept all her feelings of fear, doubt, excitement, or anticipation and be prepared to accept her parents' reactions to her news. Parents of teen mothers experience a wide range of emotions also. Research demonstrates that parents of pregnant teens often feel disappointment at themselves or with their child; they feel their dreams, hopes, and hard work have failed. They feel like they themselves are failures as parents or that they let their child down. Often a fantasy, or vision, of a perfect life, and perfect child, has been disrupted. However, whatever emotion is displayed by a teen's parents, those emotions are theirs and are not the responsibility of teen parents to address. Research further supports that despite any immediate emotions or responses most parents of pregnant teens love their children and want what is best, and safest, for them. Teen parents should embrace whatever support they receive when it is offered and forthcoming.

Teen mothers, or teen parents, need to remind themselves that they have power throughout the entire disclosure process, the pregnancy, and the childbirth process. People will treat them only how a teen mother, or teen parents, permit themselves to be treated; they should therefore project, and expect, a good outcome. Social workers or counselors can assist with developing necessary communication skills or with developing scripting to deliver the message. Sharing the truth about a pregnancy allows teen parents to create a support network with positive, and loving, interactions to promote the best outcome for the teen parents and the baby.

38. Do my parents have to be involved in any decisions I make regarding the pregnancy?

A pregnant teen, regardless of age, holds all decision-making power over themselves. For teen mothers specifically, this means only she can make decisions for what will happen to her and her baby. Regardless of how involved a teen mother's parents may be in her life, her parents cannot force or coerce her into a decision (e.g., have an abortion, put the baby up for adoption, or keep the baby), nor can they make any decisions on the teen mother's behalf after the baby is born unless a true medical emergency or other extraordinary circumstance exists. Essentially, a pregnant teen is looked on as someone who made an adult decision (i.e., have sex) and now must manage the consequences of that adult decision.

If a pregnant teen mother is still living with her parents, she is expected to abide by the rules of that household. Those rules are typically set by her parents. In some states a pregnant teen mother may require her parents' permission to have an abortion or have her parents notified if she intends to have, or has had, an abortion. The rules vary by state and are subject to change, so using a reliable resource like the Guttmacher Institute (www. guttmacher.org) or a social worker can help a teen or her family to navigate the various regulations of each state.

Parents of a pregnant teen, however, are under no additional responsibility to assist a pregnant teen mother. Aside from providing a home, food, and other basic needs for a teen mother, the parents of a teen mother are under no other obligation to care for and support the baby even though the baby is their grandchild. Depending on the age of the mother, parents can ask her to leave their home if the teen mother leaving does not pose a danger to her or the unborn baby and seek alternative living arrangements. Parents are also not obligated to pay for any expenses for the pregnant teen mother and can opt to not cover her under their insurance plan.

Most parents, however, are supportive of their pregnant teen despite the circumstances that led to the pregnancy occurring. Parents of pregnant teens become useful resources to help them navigate the multiple decisions that lie ahead for them. Further, parents role model parenting behaviors for teen parents and assist their transition to parenthood. Because most parents of pregnant teens are involved in each teen's life, it is necessary, however, for both the teens and their parents to set guidelines for what is expected of them both during pregnancy and after delivery.

During pregnancy, a teen mother has changing needs. She and her parents need to define the expectations of each one's role related to the mother's needs (e.g., health care practitioner appointments, purchase of maternity clothes, purchase items for the baby). The involvement of the father of the baby needs to also be defined. Child care, both immediately after birth and through the first years of life, also needs to be addressed.

The baby will also have changing needs after it is born. The mother and her parents will need to be clear about what is their expectations of each other especially surrounding financially supporting the baby and babysitting needs. A teen mother needs to be realistic in her plan: will she finish school or seek employment? What expenses does she think she can reasonably cover and where will she likely need assistance, either from her parents or from other support sources? Does she plan to continue living at home or start a life on her own? What will be the father of the baby's contribution toward caring for the baby? Regardless of her parents' participation, a teen mother remains the only decision maker for herself and her baby.

What is important to differentiate is a teen mother's right to make decisions for herself and her baby and any additional freedoms she may think she has. In most states, a pregnant teen is not automatically an emancipated minor. Emancipation occurs when an individual has reached the age of majority under applicable law and has the right to become independent of his or her parents' control. Age of majority, or the age at which a person is granted by law the rights (e.g., ability to sue) and responsibilities (e.g., liability under contract) of an adult; age of majority is set by a statute in each state and is 18 years of age in most states.

A minor can petition a court to become emancipated. However, there are specific conditions or circumstances that must exist for a minor to become legally responsible for themselves. Some examples include if the minor is legally married, financially independent, has abusive, neglectful, or otherwise harmful parents, or has a moral objection to their parents' living situation. In some states, however, if a pregnant teen is 16 years of age or older, she is automatically emancipated; however, emancipation is not automatic. Parents can also try to block a teen's attempt at emancipation, so the teen needs to demonstrate that she has a better chance of raising her newborn or child, and is more protected, in a household outside one with her parents.

39. Are my parents legally required to take care of me and my baby?

The parents of pregnant teens are in a unique situation: they are the responsible caretakers of underage minors and the grandparents of the baby. Although these parents are legally responsible to care for their children, they are under no obligation to care for, or support, the baby (i.e., their grandchild). However, parents' offers to help house and care for a pregnant teen or new mother and her baby are voluntary and can be revoked at any time. If a pregnant teen mother continues to reside with their parents and continues to live with them with the baby, parents or legal guardians are able to seek additional financial compensation in most states to offset the additional costs a pregnant woman or new mother and her baby will incur for the family.

Because a pregnant teen is not automatically emancipated in most states, a pregnant teen mother's parents are legally obligated to care for her, including to provide the adequate medical care she will need throughout her pregnancy. However, if a family is receiving state-funded financial assistance, it still does not convey any additional legal rights or responsibilities to the grandparents over the mother; they also continue to have no legal right to make decisions for the baby. There are few exceptions nationwide with most states having some form of statute or law requiring that parents of teen mothers continue to financially support their daughter. In some states parental support for a pregnant teen mother is mandated and may also include mandated support from the father of the baby's parents also. How that support is rendered, however, can vary, including where the source of that support originates.

Parents of a teen mother can opt to keep her on any group insurance plan that a parent may have in place (e.g., insurance provided by an employer). However, not every insurance plan has a maternity benefit, or it may not have a maternity benefit that covers the needs of pregnant dependent children. Currently, federal law does not require any insurance plan to offer or provide maternity benefit for dependent children. Further, coverage for a pregnant dependent child will not extend to, nor automatically cover, the baby. In some instances, the pregnant teen mother will need to apply for her own insurance (typically through state-funded Medicaid programs) and then use a similar program to establish insurance for her baby.

What the parents of a pregnant teen mother are not legally allowed to do is neglect her. Regardless of the circumstances surrounding a teen's pregnancy, or the parents own views related to the situation, parents cannot withhold basic needs like food and shelter from a pregnant teen mother. If a parent opts to kick their daughter out of their home, they can only do so if they have arranged safe alternative housing for her that will continue to provide her with all her basic needs. In these cases, a social worker can assist a family or a pregnant teen mother with securing safe housing and additional resources if staying with her parents is not allowed or ideal.

The father of the baby's parents may also have responsibilities to a pregnant teen mother. In most states the responsibility to support a pregnant teen mother does not fall solely to her parents. Because the father of the baby is often a teen himself and not emancipated, his parents are often obligated to share some of the financial burden for providing for a pregnant teen mother and later her baby. Like the parents of a teen mother, courts can mandate that the parents of a teen father continue to support him financially and provide some additional assistance to the teen mother. In some states the parents of a teen father may be required to pay child support after the baby is born until their son emancipates. The parents of a teen mother can also take legal action against the father of the baby's family to petition for additional support from them to support a pregnant teen mother or her baby because their own income has been jeopardized by the needs of the teen mother and her baby.

40. Do I have to get married because I'm pregnant or got someone pregnant?

Marriage is socially and culturally driven; families set the expectation whether having a child out of wedlock is acceptable. In the United States, a woman is not required to be legally married to have a baby or provide it with benefits or resources after it's born. A man who impregnates a woman outside of marriage is also under no obligation to propose marriage or marry the mother of the baby.

Marriage laws are rooted in 18th-century laws in the United States and have essentially gone unchanged. In the past, life expectancy was lower, so couples married younger or in their teen years to have their families and establish a home. Continuing education or establishing a career for men or women was largely unavailable or not a priority. At its core, marriage continues to require two people to consent to be joined in matrimony. Teenagers, however, do not have the legal capacity to provide their own consent, so many states have laws that govern when a teen is permitted to willingly consent to marriage. The age of majority is 18 in most states. Teens between the ages of 13 and 18 often require parental consent to be married. In other states, parental consent and a judge's approval are needed for teens to marry; many states, however, make it difficult for teens to marry. Even if the couple already has a child, those states still require court approval for the couple to marry.

Current research concluded that teens are ambivalent about marriage. Although most report that they expect to get married someday and that being married is a good thing, many have witnessed or known single parents who have successfully raised a child on their own. Others have also been exposed to people who postponed marriage and parenthood until later adulthood, so the impetus to marry young is missing. However, teens have also reported that they feel getting married legitimizes their relationship or the baby and takes away the stigma of being a single teen parent or the stereotype of being "bad." Teen fathers are often considered to be "manning up," "doing the right thing," or making a teen mother an "honest woman" by marrying her. However, marriage under those circumstances portrays teen mothers as totally dependent and incapable of managing parenthood alone. Motherhood for teen girls becomes a chore or a duty and not a choice.

Relationships and marriage forged during pregnancy can be unpredictable. Being pregnant can bond a couple, but it is difficult for either parent to feel romantic and emotional during pregnancy. Being pregnant and getting married does not guarantee a successful marriage or a long-term relationship. Although marriage may seem like the right thing to do for religious and social reasons, it can take an emotional, physical, and financial toll on a teen couple. Although some teen marriages are successful with the couple working through hardships and staying committed to each other, the baby, and their future family, research supports that teen marriages do not last after the first few years. Research also concluded that ill-fated marriages add further stress to both the pregnant teen mother and the couple. Marriage, with its advantages and disadvantages, is ultimately a personal decision that a teen couple needs to carefully consider.

41. What rights and responsibilities does the baby's father have?

Teen fathers have significant rights and responsibilities related to their baby. However, it is important to distinguish between a right and a responsibility. A right is a freedom that is protected under the law (e.g., in the United States, freedom of speech or a fair trial). A responsibility is a duty or something one should do, typically because it is the right thing to do. Responsibilities are things people can control and are often defined as personal, agency, or moral responsibilities. Despite the differences between each, rights and responsibilities usually go together and are often related.

Teen fathers who are not married to the pregnant teen mother, first and foremost, have the right to know if they are truly the father of the baby. Teen fathers have the right to request, or sue for, confirmation of paternity. Fatherhood is a lifelong personal and financial commitment, so teen fathers have the right to request DNA paternity testing to confirm if a baby is theirs. DNA paternity testing, however, can only occur after the baby is born.

DNA paternity testing remains the most popular method of confirming paternity. Although potentially complicated and expensive, the test can be invaluable. Some laboratories have payment plans to alleviate some of the costs associated with paternity testing. The most accurate DNA testing is done using samples from the mother, the identified father, and the child, but testing can be done with just samples from the identified father and the child. The test currently is easy and painless: a small wooden or plastic stick or a cotton-tipped applicator is used to scrape cells from the inside of each person's cheek. There is no bleeding or injury to either person, and the gentle swabbing takes only a few seconds. The DNA in the cells from each sample is then analyzed and graphed into a sequence. The DNA sequence of the child is compared to one or both parents to determine if the sequences match. The degree to which those sequences match is reported as a percentage. Thus, a 0% result means there is no chance the teen is the father of the baby, and a result of 99% (or higher including decimal positions) means the teen is the baby's father. Other results or differing percentage results often mean the tests need to be repeated.

Once paternity is confirmed or accepted, a teen father has the right to know his child and participate in his child's life. Further, a teen father has the right to custodial access to his child. Teen mothers cannot prevent a teen father from seeing, visiting, or spending time with the child unless she has valid reasons for doing so; those reasons must be approved by the courts. Teen fathers are often required to pay child support if the child does not live with them; conversely, if a teen father is raising the child, the child's mother may also be required to pay child support to the father. In most states, a teen father also has the right to restrict who sees his child and for how long, or they can restrict anyone from visiting their child. A teen father has the right to enroll his child in school and to obtain medical treatment for the child if needed. A teen father can also apply for benefits for his child, and in an emergency or other urgent situation do anything necessary a parent with legal custody can do.

A teen father has no rights when the baby is unborn, and the teen mother is pregnant. A teen father cannot stop the mother of the baby from having an abortion. Therefore, a teen father has almost no rights while the baby is in utero. However, a teen father has the right to prevent his child from being surrendered for adoption. For an adoption to take place, the teen father must sign over his rights to the child to the adoptive family. A teen mother does not have to list the father of the baby's name on the birth certificate, hence the need for confirmatory DNA paternity testing. A teen father may need to bring legal action against the baby's mother so paternity testing can be completed.

If paternity is confirmed and child support and a custody arrangement have been agreed on, a teen father has the responsibility to be a father to his child. Fatherhood responsibilities include being present in, and contributing to, his child's life. This includes knowing his child, participating in its life, and to support and care for the child by paying child support to its mother if he is not the custodial parent.

As a parent, a teen father is responsible to keep his child free from harm and that the child is well cared for. A father also provides for his child's emotional needs by supplying stability, consistency, encouragement, and interest in the child's life. A father becomes a role model, so it is essential that he carefully choose work, a social or friendship network, activities, habits, or interests that reflect positive attributes that his child can replicate. This includes spending time with the child and helping with child care. A teen father should focus on completing his education like graduating high school or obtaining a GED, attending college, or obtaining vocational training. If teen fathers feel they lack the necessary resources to be a successful parent, including adequate role models from their own childhood, various programs are available to assist teen fathers to develop themselves into good fathers. Health care practitioners, social workers, counselors, community, or religious leaders can provide direction or referral to teen fathers to find and access any needed resources.

42. Can the baby's father get custody of the baby?

For the father of the baby to have any kind of visitation or custody of the baby, he has to first acknowledge that he is the father of the baby (i.e., acknowledge paternity). If the father's name is not on the baby's birth certificate, a father can request, or sue for, a paternity test to confirm he is the father of the baby and then file an Order of Filiation with the courts. The father's name on the birth certificate, however, holds equal weight as the mother's.

Fathers are less likely to get custody of a baby or a child if the mother is deemed to be a good parent. Courts typically favor the mother having custody of a baby or child. Some mothers may volunteer to give custody of the baby to the father, but those circumstances are rare. Different types of custody exist. *Physical custody* is when the parent has the right to have a child live with him or her. Where the child lives primarily with one parent and has visitation with the other, the parent with whom the child lives (or the custodial parent) will have sole or primary physical custody, and the other parent (the noncustodial parent) will have the right to visitation or parenting time with his or her child. *Legal custody* means having the right and obligation to make decisions about a child's upbringing. A parent with legal custody can make decisions about the child's schooling, religious upbringing, and medical care. In most states, courts regularly award joint legal custody, which means important decisions about a baby or child is shared by both parents. *Sole custody* means one parent has legal and physical custody of a baby or child. In most states courts will not hesitate to award sole custody to one parent if the other parent is deemed unfit (e.g., the other parent has alcohol or drug dependency or charges of child abuse or neglect). *Joint custody* is most common where both parents do not live together but share decision-making responsibility for the baby or child. In joint custody, the baby or child spends equal or close to equal amount of time with both parents.

If a custody case is brought by either parent against the other for modifying a custody agreement, the courts try to give each parent equal opportunity to prove that he or she is the better parent for the baby or child. Courts will, overall, try to do what is in the best interest of a baby or child. Judges will consider several factors like the mental and physical health of the parents. Judges will also want to know if either parent has a history of domestic violence and what their relationships are like with other family members. How each parent is paying child support and which parent is more likely to honor visitation will also be considered.

For a father to gain physical or sole custody of a baby or child, he will have to demonstrate that the child's mother is not fit to be the custodial parent. A father will have to show a judge, mediators, lawyers, or other family court experts what happened and show the mother's consistent pattern of inappropriate behaviors. Fathers are often asked to keep a journal or upload information onto a secure database managed by his lawyer and document dates, times, and places where any inappropriate behaviors occurred. Questionable or inappropriate behaviors by a mother can include making the handoff of a baby or child for visitation and showing up late, or missing a handoff or changing the handoff location without notifying the father. Refusal to honor a father's request for more time with the baby or child or refusing to allow phone or video time with an older child can also be considered inappropriate. Acts of aggression, violence, or being confrontational, especially in the presence of the baby or child, can also be used against a mother. Any police involvement or a mother being arrested and/ or becoming incarcerated would also assist a father with gaining custody. The baby or child can also help determine custody; a child who is sad or unhappy, acts out, becomes withdrawn, or behaves differently with one parent can also impact a judge's or court's decision about custody.

43. What are the legal implications of a pregnancy caused by rape or incest?

Rape is a crime. Rape is a type of sexual violence with forced or alcohol/ drug-facilitated anal, oral, or vaginal penetration. More women are raped by a current or former partner compared to those who are raped by an acquaintance or a stranger. Hence, most women know their rapist. Of those women who are raped by a partner, 30% were forced into the sex act with 20% of those women reporting that the partner tried to get them pregnant when the woman did not want pregnancy to occur or their partner tried to prevent them from using birth control (known as reproductive coercion).

More than 15% of adolescent girls worldwide have experienced forced sexual intercourse or other sexual acts at some point in their lives. A growing number of international studies are revealing that the first sexual experience for girls is often unwelcome or forced. Sexual abuse leads to unwanted pregnancy because young or teenage girls are less likely to have the opportunity or choice to use contraception. Girls, therefore, are at the greatest risk of exposure to sexual violence within the context of a close relationship like family, friends, or an intimate partner.

A rapist uses force or violence to take control over another human being. It is about power, not sex. Rape is not the victim's fault. Rape can occur under various circumstances and may also occur in the presence of alcohol or drug intoxication. If a teenage girl is raped, her safety is the priority. Immediately after the event she should find a secure place away from the perpetrator. She should not change her clothes, shower, douche, or wash. Telling a trusted adult, or family member, would assist her in taking the next important steps. Rape crisis centers are in most cities, but a national hotline (800-656-HOPE) is available. Hospital emergency departments and clinics are also places to obtain resources and referrals to rape counselors, social workers, or advocates.

It is important to seek medical care after a rape occurs. An ideal window to have a medical evaluation completed would be within 72 hours of

the rape occurring; if more than 72 hours have passed, a medical evaluation can still be completed. Although a medical evaluation from a health
care practitioner may seem daunting after a rape, the examination will
allow a health care practitioner to do a full assessment for injuries, test for
sexually transmitted diseases, allow any needed medical care to be administered, and any evidence that could be used to prosecute the perpetrator
collected in the proper fashion. An emergency department (ED) is the
typical place to have this important examination.

ED staff provide support to a girl who has been raped. A social worker,
advocate, or counselor trained in helping rape victims is usually summoned
to provide additional support and will help guide a rape victim through
the medical evaluation. A health care practitioner or trained examiner
will perform the evaluation. The victim, however, is in complete control
of the evaluation and can refuse any part she is not comfortable with. The
medical evaluation will include tests for sexually transmitted diseases,
including HIV. Blood or saliva samples may be taken. Antibiotic medication may be given to prevent the occurrence of sexually transmitted
diseases. The health care practitioner may also offer emergency contraception, if desired, to prevent pregnancy (e.g., the drug Plan B). A gentle
pelvic examination will be done to identify any injuries to the genital
areas. Samples of hair, skin, nails, and body fluids will be taken from the
victim's clothes and body. If there is a suspicion that drugs were used (e.g.,
rohypnol, GHB, Ecstasy, or alcohol), a toxicology test will be run to identify and confirm the presence of the substances.

Teens affected by any form of sexual assault are profoundly violated. A
rape is an attack on her body, her safety, and her security. Girls or women
who have experienced rape or other sexual assault are at risk for developing post-traumatic stress disorder (PTSD), anxiety, sleep disorders, or
depression. They are also at higher risk for suicidal thoughts or actual suicide attempts. Social workers, advocates, or trained counselors can help
a rape victim manage the variety of feelings she may experience and also
help her navigate the legal process if she wishes to do so.

Some rape victims may be reluctant to call the police. There is a high
degree of fear or embarrassment about drawing attention to the violation,
or they may try to protect the perpetrator if it is someone they know.
There may also be a high degree of fear about retaliation, a repeat attack,
or further harm to herself or her family. Reporting the rape, however, is a
powerful step to protect others from the perpetrator.

Each state has a different statute of limitations that determines the
length of time a person can wait before filing changes against another
for a crime. If a woman opts to pursue legal action, she first must file a

police report. After the police report is completed, a girl or woman has the option to press charges against the perpetrator or not. If charges are filed, the case will be assigned to a detective who will perform an investigation and gather evidence, including an interview of both the victim and the perpetrator. It can take several days for the detective to gather all the necessary information. The evidence and supporting documentation will be presented to a prosecutor who will determine what charges will be filed against the perpetrator. The perpetrator will then be arrested, and he begins his defense process.

Some court cases are dropped due to lack of evidence. A preliminary hearing will be held where the evidence against the perpetrator is presented or a grand jury is convened. The prosecutor turns over the evidence to the defense attorney. This stage of the trial is usually the longest. The final stage is an actual trial where the evidence and testimony will be heard and debated. A trial culminates in a verdict of guilty or not guilty. If guilty, the perpetrator will receive a sentence that can vary in severity and length from state to state. A person convicted of rape will likely have to register as a sex offender.

However, a rape can also result in a pregnancy. Rape-related pregnancy (RRP) is a public health problem. More than 3 million women in the United States experience RRP during their lifetime. The occurrence of RRP is similar across racial and ethnic groups. Despite the violence surrounding a rape, once a man is identified as the father of the baby, he may still have certain rights surrounding his child. The rights he has differ from state to state. For example, in some states the father of baby born after an RRP may still be entitled to visitation, or he may still be required to pay child support.

Incest

Incest is defined as sexual activity between family members or close relatives. Incest can occur between blood relatives (e.g., father, mother, brother, or sister) or those related by affinity (e.g., through marriage, a stepfamily, or adoption). Like rape, incest is a crime. However, incest is defined differently in each U.S. state; it can be limited to only the occurrence of sexual activity in some states but may include sexual activity, marriage, or living together romantically in others. Incest is more likely to happen between an adult and a child or teen below the age of majority compared to the incidence of it occurring between two adults. Research confirmed that incest is widespread internationally with more than 37% of girls reporting sexual abuse or forced sexual activity from an adult close relative. Incest, however, is considered taboo internationally.

Unlike rape, which often occurs at one time, incest occurs over a period of time, repeatedly. Incest is similar to rape because it is forced sexual activity without consent or with someone who is not considered capable of giving consent. However, incest occurring over a period of time is often shrouded in a veil of embarrassment with many victims not accepting, understanding, or realizing the acts perpetrated against them are wrong. Many victims often want to maintain their privacy or fear harm or trouble coming to their perpetrator.

Laws in the United States ban intimate relationships between children and their parents, brothers, sisters, or between grandparents and grandchildren. Some states ban relationships between aunts, uncles, nieces, nephews, and cousins. Laws vary, however, for relationships between half siblings or step siblings, and adopted relatives. First, second, and third cousins are often free to marry in most states in the United States.

Like circumstances involving rape, pregnancy can also occur with incest. However, laws within the United States are often very stringent where incest is involved. Like rape, any sexual behavior against a child that is under the age of consent is classified as a forcible sex act. It does not matter the nature of consent or whom the relationship was pursued by. Incest is often punished severely in each state and, in most instances, the father of a baby conceived through an incestuous relationship has no legal right to be involved in any decision regarding the baby, nor does he have any influence on the child's upbringing. Termination of any paternal rights differs state to state.

A pregnancy that occurs because of incest is complicated. When two relatives, especially close first-degree relatives, conceive a baby, there is a high possibility that genetic disorders or defects will be transmitted to the child because the mother and father of the baby share most of the same genetic pedigree. These defects can either be passed onto the child that will be evident at birth or may develop later in life. Women who become pregnant because of incest are often offered the option to abort the pregnancy.

Aborting a baby who was conceived because of incest is often considered the compassionate thing to do. However, abortion carries its own risks and complications. Pro-life advocates argue that aborting a child that was conceived because of incest does not punish the criminal or the perpetrator but the child.

Regardless of the circumstances, incest, like rape, carries a significant emotional and psychological impact to the victim. Research confirms that incest victims suffer long-term consequences like low self-esteem, difficulties in interpersonal relationships, sexual dysfunction, and are at higher risk for mental disorders. Incest victims are also susceptible to substance abuse, post-traumatic stress disorder (PTSD), or become abusers themselves. Help is available for incest victims. Social workers, counselors, or sexual abuse counselors are a resource for victims. Treatment and recovery, however, can take many years.

44. What can happen if the mother is a minor and the father of the baby is a legal adult?

Sex with minors is illegal in most states in the United States and considered taboo internationally. Although the age of consent varies from state to state, the generally accepted age ranges from 16 to 18. When an adult (i.e., anyone over the age of 18) has sex with a minor, it is considered statutory rape. Statutory rape is defined as nonforcible sexual activity in which one individual is below the age of consent. Although considered sexual assault or sexual abuse in many states, statutory rape also implies some relationship existed, however inappropriate, between two parties. Therefore, overt force is not usually present when statutory rape occurs. However, a minor is still not considered capable to give consent for a sexual relationship with an adult.

Consensual teenage sex is common in the United States with people of different ages, including those who may be one to four years older. Because many teens engage in sexual relationships with other teens who may have crossed the milestone of their 18th birthday, few cases are prosecuted or lead to any arrest or convictions. Most cases surrounding statutory rape are brought against mature adults (i.e., those 21 years of age or older) who willingly engaged in a sexual relationship with a minor. Statutory rape laws are based on the premise that although young girls or boys may want to have sex, they may not have enough experience or the discernment to make a mature, informed decision. The laws protect young people who have less information and power than their age 18-and-over partners. For example, minors are considered less likely than adults to understand sexually transmitted diseases (STDs), have access to contraception, or have the resources to raise a child if they become pregnant. Statutory rape laws are intended to punish heinous crimes of adults taking advantage of a minor. Some jurisdictions also specify a minimum difference for the offense to be applicable. Known as the "Romeo and Juliet" laws, they serve to reduce or eliminate the penalty of the crime in cases where the couple's age difference is small and sexual contact would not have been considered rape if both partners were legally able to give consent. These laws also reduce the severity of the offense from a felony to a misdemeanor; reduce the penalty to a fine, probation, or community service; and/or eliminate the requirement that the convicted adult regis-ter as a sex offender. These laws, however, do not apply in cases of incest or if some form of an authoritative position of the older person over the younger person (e.g., teacher and student, coach and player) existed. Fur-ther, the laws would not apply if any physical force were used or if a serious physical injury occurs to the younger person.

The majority of statutory rape charges originate with the parents or guardian of the minor who is involved. Parents or guardians would notify law enforcement and file a complaint and press charges on behalf of the minor against the presumed offender. A detective will complete an inves-tigation and present the gathered facts to the prosecutor. The prosecutor determines what charges would apply and then arrest, or issue a summons to, the offender. It would then be up to the suspected offender to prove his innocence or justify the acts committed within the court system.

Depending on the state, some common professions like physicians, nurses, social workers, teachers, child care workers, clergy members, or employees of state agencies are deemed mandated reporters. Mandated reporters are professionals or workers who are required by law, based on their role, to monitor for, and report, any suspected instances of abuse, especially surrounding children, or minors. Health care practitioners who treat teens who are pregnant or infected with STDs are also included as mandated reporters. Mandated reporters may be obligated to notify child protective services, child welfare agencies, family services, or the department of social services if they suspect or discover that a teen is having sex with an adult under the statutes that govern child sexual abuse. Mandated reporters do not need proof that the abuse occurred or is occurring to make a good faith report. Further, mandated reporters do not have to disclose to the teen or parents that they are making a report to a state agency in most states.

45. Can my baby be taken away from me because I'm a teenager?

Babies, and children, are vulnerable members of society. They are com-pletely dependent on their parents, a guardian, or a caretaker for all of their basic human needs. When there is a question about, or concern for, a child's well-being, if the child is living in a safe home environment, or if a mother, parents, guardian, or caretaker is able to care for a child, Child Protective Services (CPS) is notified. CPS is a branch of a state's social services department that is responsible to assess, investigate, and intervene for suspected or actual child abuse and neglect, including sexual abuse. CPS practices vary state to state and may be called by different names or use different acronyms, but their purpose is the same: to protect children from caregivers who may be harming them. Although teen mothers have a higher incidence of substance abuse, depression, and anxiety, and lack resources like adequate housing or financial support compared to adult women, any mother or family could fall under the scrutiny of CPS if certain conditions or situations arise regardless of the age of the parent or child.

Many professions in the United States (e.g., physicians, nurses, social workers, teachers, police officers) are mandated reporters. Mandated reporters are legally obligated to report any signs of abuse or neglect of a child to the appropriate authorities like CPS immediately. CPS is legally obligated to investigate every report it receives. Investigations by CPS vary and often include interviewing the child and other siblings if possible, the parents or family, and exploring any available evidence. CPS investigations are thorough and meant to uncover patterns of behaviors, looking for areas that can be stressors for parents like relationships with domestic violence, drug or alcohol abuse, the burdens of child care, or lack of necessary resources to care for a child. Although some cases investigated by CPS are found meritless, others require intervention.

CPS strives to keep children with their parents and to keep families together. However, in some dire cases children will be removed from a dangerous environment immediately. Removal of a child requires a court order from a judge. Parents will need an attorney and are required to attend a hearing with a judge to determine the next steps for the family. In contrast, placement of a child is when a parent voluntarily gives the child temporarily to a family member or other close relative and the child stays in that person's home. In addition, children who have been removed may also have an opportunity to be placed in another family member's care. Foster care is the last resort. CPS workers attempt to exhaust every other safe option before exploring placement of a child in the foster system. Further, removal of a child does not mean that the child can never be returned to a parent's custody. CPS works with a family to provide any support, skills training, or assistance a family may need to reunite them as a whole family unit again. CPS works to improve a family, not destroy it. Permanent, nonvoluntary termination of parental rights is a complicated process that is reserved for only the most extreme cases of abuse or neglect.

❖

Other Concerns

46. What do I do if I don't know who the father is?

Teenage girls, and adult women, who engage in a monogamous relationship, or who are only having sex with one man, know immediately who the father of their baby is. However, girls or women with multiple sex partners may not be certain who the father of the baby could be. A woman's menstrual cycle may be useful to assist her to identify who the baby's father could be.

If a woman has menstrual periods that are regular, she can likely calculate when she was most fertile and likely, then, to conceive. Most women with regular cycles ovulate about 2 weeks before the first day of their period, even if their cycles are shorter or longer than the typical 28 days. Therefore, if a woman knows when her period was due, she can count back 2 weeks to find an ovulation date. That date is when she most likely conceived. If a woman had sex in the 5 days before ovulation, there is a strong chance that sperm cells were still alive in the vagina or cervix and ready to fertilize an egg when it was released. However, if a woman had more than one sexual partner during her most fertile time, it may be difficult for her to know for certain which partner is the baby's father.

Women with irregular periods may have more difficulty narrowing down the date she conceived. For women with unreliable, inconsistent periods she may have to wait for her first ultrasound examination. Between 10 to 13 weeks an ultrasound can determine how many weeks pregnant a woman is and predict the date the baby is due to be born. Once a woman has a due date calculated by ultrasound, she can count back 38 weeks to give her an opportunity to try to identify who her sexual partners were at that time. There are various applications (i.e., apps) for handheld devices that also try to pinpoint dates of conception, but ultrasound remains the most accurate form of technology compared to counting from the first day of the last period. If a woman still cannot determine who the father of her baby is, she may have to wait until delivery of the baby to determine paternity. There are tests that can be done during pregnancy, but they carry the risk of miscarriage so they are often discouraged. A paternity test after delivery is recommended with each potential father.

Every child has a biological father. If a baby is born to a woman who is married, her husband is automatically listed as the baby's father in most states in the United States. When a child is born to unmarried parents, the child has no legal father, and the biological father has no rights or responsibilities to the child. However, a woman cannot simply put a man's name of the baby's birth certificate and claim he is the father of the baby. Unmarried parents can establish paternity by signing a form where a man voluntarily accepts paternity of the baby; the mother or father can also petition the court to establish paternity. The court will, typically, order the mother, child, and alleged father to submit to certain genetic tests. Based on the results of the testing, the court will determine whether the alleged father is the legal father of the child. If the alleged father is shown to be the biological father, the court will issue an Order of Filiation declaring that the man is the father of the child.

47. How does a paternity test work?

Deoxyribonucleic acid (DNA) is the molecule that contains the genetic code of organisms. This includes animals, plants, and humans. DNA is in each cell in the organism and tells the cells what proteins to make. These proteins are mostly enzymes. DNA is inherited by children from their parents. Thus, DNA in a person is a combination of the DNA from each of their parents. Because DNA is unique, paternity testing involves looking at DNA profiles to determine whether an individual is the biological parent of another individual. Further, DNA testing can be used to determine the likelihood that someone is the biological grandparent of an individual. There are multiple ways to obtain DNA and determine paternity.

During the prenatal period there are some ways to determine paternity before the baby is born. Noninvasive prenatal paternity (NIPP) testing is the most accurate way to establish paternity before the baby is born. This test analyzes the baby's DNA found naturally in the mother's bloodstream. This test requires only a simple blood collection from the mother and the alleged father. It can be performed any time after the eighth week of pregnancy. However, NIPP can be a costly test. Because it is not a medical necessity, most insurance plans do not cover the cost of NIPP, so a parent or couple would have to pay for the test themselves.

Amniocentesis is an invasive test performed in the second trimester between the 14th and 20th weeks of pregnancy. During an amniocentesis, an ultrasound is used to guide a small, thin, hollow needle into the uterus through the abdominal wall to obtain a sample of amniotic fluid. The DNA in the amniotic fluid can be compared against the alleged father's. However, amniocentesis carries significant risks like vaginal bleeding or miscarriage, so it is used only for specific circumstances.

Like amniocentesis, chorionic villi sampling is an invasive test where a thin needle is inserted into the uterus guided by ultrasound to obtain chorionic villi. The chorionic villi are finger-like projections of tissue attached to the wall of the uterus; the chorionic villi and the fetus come from the same fertilized egg and have the same genetic makeup. This testing can be done as early as 10 to 13 weeks of pregnancy.

Most paternity testing occurs after a baby is born. DNA testing remains the most advanced and accurate technology to determine parentage. Paternity testing after a baby is born is affordable, painless, and easy. Since DNA is present in most of the body's cells, a small sample for testing can be obtained from several body sources; the cells most commonly tested are from blood samples or from cells inside the cheek in the mouth called buccal cells. Testing cells from inside the cheek is a simple, painless process. A cotton swab is gently rubbed along the inside of the cheek to collect cell samples from the alleged father and from the child. The swab is sent to a laboratory where a number of DNA sequences are examined to determine if the DNA collected from the baby match the DNA collected from the alleged father. Results of DNA paternity testing from cheek swabs are usually available within 5 to 10 days.

Several at-home DNA paternity test kits have been developed that can be purchased over the Internet or in select retail stores or pharmacies. The at-home kit contains all the necessary materials and instructions for conducting a cheek cell DNA swab test. After the cheek cells are collected, the sample is sent to the laboratory for analysis. If the test is done correctly according to the product instructions, privately conducted home tests do not differ from a test required by a court order. However, for court-ordered testing the alleged father must report to a designated testing facility so the testing can be witnessed and fingerprints or identity of the donor confirmed. Without legal identification of the test taker and official witnessing of the test, a home paternity test is not admissible in court.

Costs for paternity testing vary. Tests can be as low as $100 for home test kits to over $500 for the complete testing process through an accredited facility. Prenatal paternity testing, however, is very expensive because of the need for additional equipment and physician fees to perform the test.

48. Will people be able to tell that I'm pregnant?

The growing baby inside a woman causes the uterus, as an organ, to enlarge and expand. That growth gives a woman the telltale sign of pregnancy, commonly called the "baby bump" or simply "the bump." Known as the gravid abdomen, the growth and size of a woman's abdomen is indicative of the baby's well-being and growth pattern. Health care practitioners will use measuring tape to assess the distance in centimeters of the growing pregnant abdomen from the pubic bone to the top of the uterus; the expectation is that after 24 weeks of pregnancy the measurement in centimeters should equal the week of pregnancy plus or minus 2 centimeters.

From the moment of conception to about the 12th week of pregnancy, the uterus grows but remains an organ within the pelvis. After 12 weeks, the growing uterus begins to rise up and out of the pelvis, giving a woman a small protrusion at the pubic bone. By the 16th to 20th week of pregnancy, the top of the uterus is often visible at the belly button. With each week, the uterus will continue to grow and protrude forward. At the end of the third trimester the baby begins to settle lower and starts to navigate its way into the birth canal; the pregnant abdomen "drops," and the roundness of the abdomen is more focused in the lower abdomen or pelvis instead of under or close to the ribs.

Because each woman's body, and each pregnancy, is different, women show their pregnancy differently. "Showing" occurs at different intervals for women also. Most women who begin to show early are often bloated;

bloating is caused by the sudden increase in hormones early in pregnancy that causes abdominal distention that can be mistaken for an enlarging uterus. Increasing intake of fiber and fluids can help decrease bloating. The position of the uterus can also affect how soon a woman begins to show. A uterus that is tilted toward the back could take longer to show during the early months of pregnancy compared to a uterus that tilts toward the front. Women who have had previous pregnancies, previous abdominal surgery, or who are carrying more than one baby will also likely show that they are pregnant sooner. Tall, slender women will often have more noticeable abdominal growth than obese women. Most women can reliably expect to have a visible, growing abdomen by 12 to 16 weeks of pregnancy.

Although many women are excited about their growing abdomen as an announcement about being pregnant, not every woman embraces having her pregnancy be visible. Most women have only a brief window to conceal their pregnancy. To mask their growing abdomen, women should avoid tight-fitting clothes that hug the abdominal area and opt for loose-fitting dresses, blouses, or shirts. Layering with jackets and sweaters or wearing clothes with thicker fabrics like cable knit in appropriate weather or climates can also disguise a growing abdomen. Fashion experts further recommend that empire-waisted items that cinch under the breasts provide a natural silhouette. Wearing black or dark colors, alone or in combination, can also hide the abdominal area. Pairing loose items with form-fitting items makes clothes look proportional. Women are also advised to avoid tucking tops into pants. Tops with a lot of detail at the neck, or using earrings or bold, large necklaces draws attention away from the abdomen and up to the face. Scarves and shawls in appropriate climate and weather can also add draping. Hats or sunglasses can also draw attention up to the face and away from the abdomen.

Women who want to avoid wearing or purchasing maternity clothes can engineer their regular clothing to still make it wearable. Pants can be held together using a hair tie, ponytail holder, or thick rubber band at the button and loop closure. Pants can also be left unbuttoned, and a belly band or abdominal support binder can be used to hold the top of the pants in place. A long shirt should cover the top of the pants. Women are advised to avoid certain positions that would expose their abdomen like lying down or bending over. Women should opt for side-lying positions with a pillow in front of them for support and use a chair or table for support when bending and squat using their knees. A large purse or bag can also be carried in front of their body to shield a view of the abdomen.

49. Will my pregnancy affect my current or future relationships?

Pregnancy can change a teen parent's relationship with their partner. Some people cope with these changes easily, but some find it harder. Pregnancy hormones can make a teen mother feel a mix of emotions that can make her feel vulnerable and anxious. Some teen mothers also have trouble coping with their symptoms and, coupled with any complications they might be having in the pregnancy, can cause extra stress. A positive relationship, however, can provide a teen mother or parent with feelings of love and support that can enable them to deal with their feelings.

Couples argue. It is normal for teen couples to argue even in the most healthy relationship. Couples often argue because of stress, feeling sick, or because of feeling anxious, worried, or frustrated. Pregnancy can change a couple, and the transition from being a couple to being parents is not easy. Teen couples are advised to discuss their feelings openly and honestly and to talk about what causes them anxiety. Specifically, teen parents should discuss their hopes, fears, expectations about life after the baby, the kind of parents they hope to be, and how each parent thinks they can support the other. Sometimes problems in a relationship can seem overwhelming. Some teens may feel like they are dealing with everything on their own and feel isolated or resentful. Teens, or teen couples, who feel unhappy may find that talking through their problems is helpful. However, some couples who are expecting a baby may still split up.

Teens who become pregnant tend to be in an intimate relationship that becomes less serious, or break up, at the time of the pregnancy. These relationships continue to deteriorate after pregnancy and are often violent before, or become violent after, pregnancy. Most teen mothers, however, are involved with other men who did not father their baby. Research demonstrates that teen girls who could have avoided pregnancy in their unfavorable, unstable relationship would have been in a potentially better relationship instead. Splitting up, especially while pregnant, can be devastating for a couple, especially for the pregnant teen mother. Despite a breakup, teen mothers are still entitled to financial and housing support, and additional funds to help her raise the baby.

One issue with teen couples who try to stay together despite the hardship an impending pregnancy may cause is the reality of domestic violence. Domestic violence can take many forms, including physical, sexual, emotional, psychological, or financial abuse. One in four women experience domestic abuse or domestic violence at some point in their lives. Some abuse, however, begins when a woman is pregnant. Other times the abuse gets worse during or after pregnancy. Domestic violence not only causes emotional and mental health problems like stress or anxiety but also can put an unborn child at risk. It may be difficult for a teen mother to recognize that she is being abused; however, help is available to all women that is confidential.

Following the birth of a baby, relationships change for teen parents in the future. If the relationship between the teen parents is unsuccessful, each parent will have the opportunity to date other people and potentially develop other long-lasting, intimate relationships. The major difference for teen parents is that they can no longer date freely; the needs of the baby or child will dictate how much time, energy, and money a teen or young adult may have to dedicate to meeting someone new and toward spending time with them. Balancing other responsibilities, like completing school and maintaining a home or a job, can be difficult.

Most teen parents have joint custody of the child, so it is possible to date when there is free time. However, many teens find that there are not many people who want to date someone who is also dealing with the challenges of being a parent. Many teen mothers report having a baby is a strike against them, making them a lesser woman or a less desirable person to date. Some studies have shown that the responsibility of raising a child takes away from the fun and spontaneity of dating. Teen girls have reported that the pool of eligible men or boys to date is dramatically smaller than before pregnancy, with many boys or young men not mature enough to understand what being a parent entails. Further, potential partners are not comfortable competing with a child for attention or time, with the child invariably coming first. Teen boys and young men have also verbalized that they never intended to raise another man's child or get involved in any argument or disagreements between the baby's mother and father.

Teen girls who resume dating after having a baby report that they felt rushed and pressured to please men who appeared to be worthy companions. Teen boys and young men reported that potential dates thought that a teen mother would be more "easy" and that sex was more likely to happen with girls who had already had children. Teen girls, similarly, reported having sex more often and more freely, verbalizing that men assumed that girls who had given birth were more accustomed to sexual activity. Other teen girls report that having a baby gave them a new sense of maturity and responsibility, something teen boys or young men their age are often lacking. Teen girls report dating older men because they understood the responsibilities and complexities of balancing child care, home, work, and achieving personal goals like completing their education.

A single lifestyle can be detrimental to one's emotional, mental, and physical health. Studies demonstrate that loneliness has serious effects comparable to cigarette smoking or obesity. Further, one can be surrounded by family and friends and still feel lonely. Romantic relationships, even those that are casual and not serious or committed, can provide a needed outlet for physical contact and adult communication. Long periods without dating, perhaps due to the demands of parenthood, school, or work can sometimes drive a teen to move quickly into relationships they do start. However, jumping straight into a serious exclusive relationship can be harmful, especially if it is with the wrong person.

Dating, and sustaining meaningful relationships, can be difficult for anyone. Teen parents, however, face additional challenges and require more from potential partners like honesty, dependability, patience, kindness, and flexibility. Teen parents should be assured that there are suitable partners in the world for them, but they just might be a little more difficult to find.

50. Will my social life change because I'm pregnant?

Pregnancy changes a teen mother's social circle and her normal social activities. Research demonstrates that pregnant teens often become distant from friends and no longer feel part of a social circle especially if she is the first, or only, member of a group to become pregnant or have a baby. Other research supports that, regardless of age, 50% of women reported that they lost contact with a group of their friends after becoming pregnant, and 25% of women admitted that their time available to meet up with friends and be social was diminished due to pregnancy. Many women and teen girls felt they were rejected by their group of friends.

Psychotherapists, however, explain this rejection as behavior that is based on jealousy because the other friends are not in the same position as the pregnant mother. Regardless of the circumstances surrounding the pregnancy, other girls or women do not want to be reminded of a path they are not taking or of a major life experience they are being denied. Friends, or the social circle, become irritated that a key member of their group cannot participate in all the activities of the group, so the easiest thing to do is exclude her. However, teen mothers have an opportunity to redefine themselves and their friendships. Real friendships tend to become readily apparent during a time of turmoil or uncertainty like a teen pregnancy. True friends will remain and be supportive regardless of a pregnant teen's physical discomforts or limitations.

Psychologists recommend that pregnant teens look at the situation from their friends' or social circle's perspective. People who are not parents or pregnant may not fully grasp the magnitude of what a pregnant teen mother is dealing with. Friends may be offering a teen mother space to sort out her feelings or necessary details for her life with a baby. Pregnancy is also a time for teen mothers to make new friends, including other girls or women who are in a similar situation. Studies demonstrate that new friendships formed during pregnancy are often strong and develop a "circle of trust" among girls or women who are sharing a similar situation.

Teen girls and women are advised to try to keep in contact with their circle of old friends throughout pregnancy. Although pregnancy is a time of great change, after the birth of the baby old friends remain important in a person's life. Although maintaining those friendships may seem difficult, there are ways for teen mothers to compromise and invite their friends into activities they can all share and that do not revolve around unhealthy activities like drinking or excessive partying. For example, teen mothers can invite their friends to join them for a walk, lunch, or time together watching television or a movie.

Teen mothers and parents may need to accept that some of their friendships will change because of the pregnancy and becoming a parent. Many teen parents worry that they will never have fun or go out again. Although spending time with friends may not be as spontaneous or frequent after pregnancy as it was before, it is still possible to maintain a social life. It may take additional planning, but pregnancy can be an ideal time to solidify and strengthen relationships with old friends and new friendships also.

When the baby arrives, it can be an overwhelming and emotional time. Sleep deprivation and the anxiety of being a new parent can also diminish a teen parent's desire to go out and be social. New parents should let their friends know when they are ready for visitors. They should also be honest and open with their friends, and family, about how they feel or how they are coping. Take friends up on offers to help with errands or to help care for the baby. Once life has settled down, it is good for parents to spend time away from the baby and share time with friends. A teen couple may also appreciate friends or family babysitting so they can enjoy time or time out with friends.

51. What do I do if my parents kick me out of the house?

Parents of teens, regardless of the circumstances, cannot simply take housing away from their children. Parents who do so place their child or teen in significant danger. However, parents can opt to not have their teen, including a pregnant teen or teen parent, live in their home any longer, but they are obligated to coordinate and arrange an alternative, safe housing arrangement for teens under 18 years of age. Further, they are obligated to continue to provide some form of financial assistance. Various circumstances, however, surround teens getting kicked out of the home.

Most times when a teen is kicked out of the home it is done so in anger, following an argument or an emotionally charged situation. The parent feels that the problem or issue will be solved, or disappear, if the teen is no longer present in the home or that revoking the privileges of living in the parent's home is punishment for behavior. Often after a cooldown period families reunite, apologize, and reestablish their relationship. However, when situations within the home pose a threat to a teen, their first priority is to go to a safe place.

Parents will make it known to a teen that he or she will no longer be living in their home and give the teen a window of time to find alternative housing arrangements. Although not ideal, this is the safest option and provides a teen time to access resources and carefully plan their next steps. Teens can contact guidance counselors, the school's health office, social workers, their health care practitioner, or trusted adult family members or friends for assistance.

If adult family or friends live close, teens are encouraged to reach out to them. The teen should ask if they would be willing to let them stay in their home until its either safe to return home again or until alternative housing arrangements can be found. Family members or other trusted adults may also serve as a neutral party or negotiator to help bring about resolution of the conflict.

Going to the police may be an option to ask for help. Police, however, must do what is legally allowed, and safe, so they may utilize resources to establish housing for a teen in need that may or may not include foster care. Although foster care may not be ideal, it is a viable option for shelter, food, and the ability to continue to attend school or make future plans. Living on the streets, however, is extremely dangerous for people of all ages, especially teens. Being homeless and pregnant poses significant risk for harm to both the mother and her baby. Organizations like the National Runaway Switchboard (800-RUNAWAY or 800-786-2929) work to keep runaway or homeless youth in the United States safe and off the streets. Hospital emergency departments can also be a temporary, safe place to go to access additional resources.

Many states have resources for people who find themselves suddenly homeless, including pregnant teens or parents. States rely on the expertise of social workers or case workers to help navigate their resource system. Options may include access to meals, shelters, or medical care if needed. Social workers can also connect teens with government-funded support programs like food stamps or food banks.

Being a pregnant teen or a pregnant teen couple is stressful, and the additional stress of no housing or disagreements with a family can become overwhelming. It is important for teens to remain positive and focused on developing themselves to be good parents. Many families regret the arguments they may have had or the actions they may have taken. Forgiveness or acceptance may come in time, but it does not change what has occurred. Counseling or support groups may be able to assist teens or families to repair their relationship and create a new one for the future.

52. Can I quit school and get a job?

In most states, the law mandates that children must attend school until the age of 16. Teens who intentionally miss school for unjustified, unauthorized, or illegal reasons from compulsory education are considered truant. Although truancy laws differ in each state, each school defines their specific policies regarding truancy. Schools are required to keep attendance records for students each day the school is open. Students who are repeatedly absent without acceptable justification and an alternative plan for schooling (e.g., homeschooling with a tutor) are reported to the state or local education department. In some schools truancy may result in the student not being able to graduate or to receive credit for classes attended until the time lost to truancy is made up through any combination of detention, fines, or summer school.

In the United States, truancy regulations are usually enforced by school officials under the context of parental responsibility. Parents are required by law to enroll their children in school and ensure the child attends school up to a certain age (typically 16 to 18) unless an absence is formally excused by a school official or the child is expelled. Some states impose significant fines on parents if their children do not attend school. In other states, parents may face short-term jail sentences. Furthermore, some states can fine, arrest, and jail parents who do not enroll their child in an acceptable, state-approved alternative learning program because of truancy. Children who are homeschooled and children enrolled in private school, however, are exempt from attending mandatory public schooling.

While truancy is the intentional act of teens missing or avoiding school, dropping out of school is when a student quits school before he or she graduates. This can include high school, college, or a university. In the United States most states allow for the ability of a teen to drop out of school without parental consent at the age of 16. However, teens should not simply stop attending school; not notifying guidance counselors or other school authorities can be counted as truancy, and any subsequent fines or other legal actions could be incurred by the teen's parents or guardian. It is best to formalize the exit process from the school.

Teens opt to drop out of school for various reasons. Drug and alcohol addiction and abuse is one of the leading causes for teens to abandon schooling. However, teens also lose interest in classes if the school environment is not stimulating or if the school does not offer classes that match the teen's interests. Some teens feel that school is unnecessary and that they would be better off making money, becoming famous, or traveling. Poverty and economic hardships can also cause teens to drop out of school and seek work. Some teens need to care for sick or older relatives, siblings, or their own children and are unable to attend school and balance family commitments. Often the school environment becomes too stressful or unsafe, especially if teens are bullied or experiencing violence, leaving teens to abandon their education. Teens who do not get along with teachers, school officials, or other school staff may opt to stop going to school. Students with special needs, psychiatric problems, physical handicaps, or disorders like attention-deficit/hyperactivity disorder (ADHD) or dyslexia may find the school environment too overwhelming, stressful, and unsupportive and opt to leave. Pregnant teens often have physical discomforts and complications, or social embarrassment about being pregnant, that prevent them from completing school. The demands of raising a baby, and child care, can make a teen opt to negate going to school and possibly seek employment.

An alarming number of students are dropping out of school to work. Most high school dropouts are typically male and Hispanic and more likely to end their education at the middle, or close to the end, of high school. There are laws, however, that govern the type and amount of work a teen can obtain. Federal laws like the Fair Labor Standards Act (FLSA) set wage, hours worked, and safety requirements for minors under the age of 18. In general, FLSA sets 14 as the minimum age for employment and limits the number of hours worked by minors under the age of 16. The FLSA also prohibits minors from working in jobs deemed hazardous (e.g., excavating, mining, driving heavy machinery). Some exceptions may exist if teens are working for their parent or guardian in their family's business. Each state, further, has their own laws that govern employment of minors; when the state law and the FLSA overlap, the law that is more protective of the minor will apply.

Jobs for teens, especially for those with limited education or vocational training, are limited. Full-time jobs for teens are difficult to find. Jobs like restaurant work, construction or general labor, cleaning homes or buildings, or other low-paying employment are common for teens. Teens get paid at least the federal minimum wage, but wages vary state to state. Most teens, however, earn less money compared to adults yet contribute more than 20% to their total household income. Teens' work hours are also limited, including how many hours a teen can work each day, depending on their age. Teens 14 to 15, for example, have more restrictions than older teens. Teens 16 and older have no limits on the amount of hours they work; those teens under 18, however, cannot work in a job that is deemed hazardous by the U.S. Department of Labor.

53. Will I be able to finish school if I have a baby?

A high school diploma, or evidence of completing high school–level education, is important. Opportunities for employment are limited for anyone who does not possess evidence that they completed high school. Pregnancy should not hinder a teen girl, or a teen parent, from attending school and earning a diploma. Public schools cannot legally expel or deny access to any student because of pregnancy or parenting. Unless a pregnant teen has strict health care practitioner's orders to not physically attend traditional school (e.g., because of the development of pregnancy complications), there is no reason why a teen cannot continue to attend school. Being at school can be difficult for a pregnant mother because she may need to miss classes if she feels sick, or she may feel embarrassed or self-conscious of her growing size or the circumstances surrounding her pregnancy to properly focus on, or participate in, her classes. If a teen is unable to attend school the traditional way (i.e., attending classes inside a school building), many schools are developing innovative ways for pregnant or parenting teens to attend schools using technology.

Some public school systems, like the San Francisco Unified School District, the St. Paul, Minnesota, and city of Chicago public school systems, have developed unique programs for pregnant or parenting teens. Intended to keep pregnant or parenting teen mothers, or teen parents, in school and to help promote their ongoing education to graduate, these programs utilize social workers to coordinate the school-based program for teens. Social workers focus on determining any barriers to education and work with outside resources to minimize those barriers. The goal of these programs is to prevent teen mothers or parents from dropping out of high school. These programs are typically small and housed within an existing high school. They collaborate with outside community agencies to provide additional support or resources. Most of these programs offer on-site health care, prenatal care, or child care services. There is usually on-site individual counseling and mentoring and both on- and off-site group or couple's therapy services. Case management services are also available to help teens navigate the multiple services they will need as parents. Staff working in these programs is intentionally diverse. Staff act as positive role models and mentors and may include academic teachers, social workers, counselors, or nurses. These programs also provide holistic education for teen mothers or parents and provide support for teens to become parents along with career counseling or preparation for future employment. These programs have demonstrated an increased rate of teen parents remaining in, and graduating from, high school. They also provide teens an opportunity to build self-confidence and increase self-esteem, improve decision-making abilities, and develop life skills. Although these innovative programs have demonstrated their efficacy and value to keep pregnant or parenting teens in high school, not every public, or private, school system is equipped to handle the special needs of these teens. Alternative education that offers scheduling and learning flexibility may be necessary to meet the needs of pregnant and parenting teens. These options include homeschooling, residential programs, or distance and online learning.

Homeschooling for high school is an acceptable and respected alternative to traditional education. Each state has different regulations that determine what is needed for successful homeschooling. Record keeping and documentation of the teen's progress is essential to meet established program goals. Homeschooling does not mean a teen's parent has to teach every course; the expansion of technology allows parents to outsource subjects, topics, or content to experts as needed. Standardized curricula for high school courses are available for parents or families. Parents who homeschool may also be able to take advantage of virtual high school platforms or online classes that are available in most states. Some teens may also be eligible to earn dual credit and earn college credits for subjects they are studying while homeschooled.

Residential programs are short-term, intensive programs for teens to receive required high school content. These programs are meant to be brief;

they provide all the necessary content for a high school curriculum over only a few weeks. School days are often several hours long, and classes are short but frequent. Most residential programs are a significant distance away from a teen's home and connected with a private school. These programs can be costly. Further, the longer class days can be overwhelming for a pregnant teen, so this option needs to be carefully explored and considered.

In recent years many programs have been developed that help a teen finish their education online. Many of these programs are low cost or tuition-free. Examples of these programs include Connections Academy, Penn Foster, Smart Horizons Careers Online High School, or James Madison High School Online. Many of these programs offer year-round, open enrollment and have diploma programs in a variety of courses.

A GED, often called the graduate equivalency degree, graduate equivalency diploma, general education diploma, or traditionally the general education development test, is a way for students to validate completion of required courses for high school. The GED is a series of tests that will indicate whether or not a person has a high school–level of education. The GED tests four main areas: mathematical reasoning, reasoning through language arts, science, and social studies. Four separate tests make up the GED, and each test is about 1 to 2 hours long. A certain score must be achieved to pass each test; each test must be passed for a GED to be granted. Passing the GED will enable a teen to earn a state high school diploma and recognition that they have a high school–level education. The GED is recognized and accepted by nearly all U.S. colleges, universities, and employers.

To take the GED exam, a teen cannot be enrolled in high school and must be at least 16 years of age. The GED exam is administered in person at a designated testing center. Each state has multiple certified testing locations. Scheduling a test is often done online. Many state, community, or local school boards offer GED preparation classes, and there are multiple books or online resources that offer practice tests, study questions, or test previews.

Teen mothers and parents should be helped to finish their high school education. For teens who have become parents, child care is often the largest obstacle to their completing high school. Day care within the high school provides mothers or teen parents the opportunity to continue their education while helping to decrease the propensity for teen mothers or parents to drop out of high school to care for children. On-site child care or day care in high schools is an innovative program to assist teens. Teens bring their child to school with them and drop the child off with qualified child care workers in the school. The teen attends classes as they normally would and then picks their child up at the end of the school day. Although various models of these programs have demonstrated their value and efficacy across the United States, opponents of these programs emphasize how costly they are for a school or a school district's budget. These are often the first programs, then, to be cut or scaled back during times of economic hardship. Opponents instead favor targeted education for teens regarding abstinence or safe sex practices.

54. Will I be able to go to college if I have a baby in my teens?

Teen pregnancy is a leading cause of school dropout among female students. Teen parents are also one of the most at-risk group of students when it comes to giving up on college. Although teen parents face real obstacles when it comes to completing their education, especially going to college, it is still possible for teen parents to graduate high school and continue their education at the college level. Becoming a parent as a teen creates serious risks, however, for their educational future. While 51% of teen mothers have a high school diploma, less than 2% of teen mothers attain a college degree by age 30. Child care, the demands of a family, and the need to work have been identified as obstacles that anyone, especially teen parents or younger adults, can face when attempting to attend college.

It is important for teen parents to recognize the challenges they may face so they can seek alternatives or solutions. Realistic goals, and a realistic time line, need to be created that will afford a teen parent or younger adult the opportunity to attend college while accommodating their child's or family's needs. Community, state, or federal resources may be available to assist a parent to create a budget and work plan to afford college.

A traditional college environment with long hours on campus or living in student dorms is not likely to work for a teen parent. Therefore, teen parents may need to consider more practical options when choosing a school. Because child care can be the biggest barrier to attending college for a parent, some schools offer on-site child care to enrolled students. For those schools without a child care option, a parent may need to stay closer to home to utilize a support system of family or friends to assist with child care. Parents also need to explore colleges that offer evening and weekend classes or self-paced degree programs to allow them to both work and attend school. If a suitable college cannot be found locally, distance or online degree programs have increased that offer a variety of affordable, flexible options for parents. Thus, applying to the right type of college or program can help increase a parent's success.

Different types of programs and educational paths exist. Cooperative education is a structured method of combining classroom-based education with practical work experience. Commonly called a "co-op," these programs provide academic credit for structured job experience. Co-ops alternate semesters of on-campus study with semesters of full-time employment. The co-op program is designed to complement a student's formal education with paid work experience that is directly related to the student's academic major. The co-op allows students to take on increasing levels of responsibility and to use their job knowledge and classroom learning. Many co-op graduates are hired by their co-op employer. Different co-op models exist, but most are found in high schools or undergraduate colleges and universities.

Vocational, or trade, schools are designed to provide technical skills required to complete tasks of a particular, and specific, job. These programs are ideal for students who are looking to directly enter the workforce because, unlike colleges and universities, the focus is on job-specific training rather than theoretical or academic education in a professional discipline. In the United States, vocational schools are often government owned or government supported. Vocational schools often require a high school diploma or a GED to enter and are typically one to two years in length. After completion of a vocational program, credits obtained for the course of study are likely to be accepted by a college or university if a student wishes to continue their education and achieve a formalized college degree.

Community colleges, also called junior or technical colleges, are two-year public institutions that grant certificates, diplomas, or associate degrees. Community colleges attract and accept students from the local community and are typically supported by local tax revenue. Admission requirements are less stringent than colleges or universities; many have open enrollment. Class schedules are flexible to meet the needs of adult learners. After graduating from community college, many students transfer to a four-year liberal arts college for an additional two to three years to complete a bachelor's degree.

Four-year colleges and universities are traditional higher education institutions. Colleges are often smaller institutions that emphasize undergraduate education in a broad range of academic areas. Universities are typically larger institutions that offer a variety of both undergraduate and graduate degree programs. Admission to a college or university typically requires a high school diploma or GED, certain coursework completed at the high school level, and often evidence of passing a standardized aptitude test like the SAT or ACT. A majority of colleges or universities waive the standardized aptitude test score submission for individuals over age 25. Some schools that do not require SAT or ACT scores for adult admission may require them, however, if a student is pursuing school-based financial aid. Completed high school course work needed for admission usually includes four years of English, three years of mathematics, a foreign language, and a science with one of those years being a laboratory science, and one year of social studies or history.

The application process for a college or university may also include an essay from the student, letters of reference or recommendation, a résumé, a transcript from high school or any other schools attended, and a fee. Students who take college courses or who previously earned college credits from coursework in high school may be able to put them toward a degree at another institution. Those students are considered transfer students, and different admission requirements exist for students transferring credits.

❖❖❖

Case Studies

1. ALYSSA DECIDES TO HAVE AN ABORTION

Alyssa is a 15-year-old high school sophomore. Alyssa is enrolled in honors courses and is also on the field hockey team. She works as a babysitter for a few hours after school and sometimes on weekends. Alyssa's parents divorced several years ago, and she lives with her mother and younger sister. On the weekends when she is not working, she often sees her father.

Alyssa has a large circle of friends that include both boys and girls of different ages in her high school. She describes herself as a shy person who has difficulty meeting, and starting conversations with, boys. Alyssa dated someone briefly but remains single through most of sophomore year to focus on her schoolwork, sports, and her babysitting job.

On a Friday night Alyssa was invited to a friend's home. When other students found out there were no adults at the home, some brought beer or whatever alcohol they could easily take from their own homes. Alyssa had never drunk alcohol before but was eager to see what drinking would be like. Throughout the evening she had finished two cans of beer and a full plastic cup of an unknown alcohol mixed with fruit juice. Alyssa began to feel the effects of the alcohol and was enjoying herself at the party.

Alyssa found herself easily talking with people at the party, especially with boys. She struck up a conversation with a boy she always thought was cute, and the two quickly advanced to kissing and touching. The two went to a secluded part of the house and, as her excitement grew, Alyssa had oral and vaginal sex with the boy.

Over the next several days Alyssa was embarrassed by what she had done. She saw the boy at school, but he avoided her and pretended like nothing happened. Alyssa was hurt but opted to put the event behind her and told no one about what happened. However, the following month Alyssa's menstrual period was late. Because Alyssa's periods were often irregular, she waited to see if it would eventually arrive. By the second month without her period, she became worried.

Alyssa feared telling her parents. Instead she went to her high school's health office and confided to the nurse what had happened. The nurse supported Alyssa and referred her to a clinic where she could get a pregnancy test and any other help she needed. At the clinic, Alyssa had a complete health history and physical examination, including STD testing, by a health care practitioner. A pregnancy test done at the clinic confirmed Alyssa was pregnant. The health care practitioner discussed Alyssa's options, including to have the baby and keep it or put it up for adoption or to have an abortion.

Alyssa needed time to analyze her choices. She dreamed that one day she would marry and have a family but anticipated that would happen in her late twenties. She barely knew the boy she had sex with and did not envision a future with him. Alyssa's parents had an unfriendly relationship after their divorce, and Alyssa did not feel comfortable telling either one of them. She knew she was not ready to become a mother and that she lacked the financial, family, and social resources she would need to raise a child. She believed having a baby would impact her ability to finish high school and possibly prevent her from going to college. An abortion, then, seemed like her only option.

Alyssa returned to the clinic and scheduled the abortion. Alyssa lives in a state that does not require parental permission or notification about the abortion. The procedure went smoothly; she was given some mild sedatives and was comfortable throughout the procedure. She had mild cramping after and only minimal bleeding. She rested for a few days and felt normal. During a follow-up visit, the health care practitioner reviewed Alyssa's progress and verified that she was not experiencing any complications. The health care practitioner had a lengthy conversation about birth control and offered to start Alyssa on oral contraceptive pills (OCPs). Alyssa declined but accepted a supply of free condoms.

Analysis

Alyssa is like many high school teenagers throughout the United States. She is a good student, plays sports, and works to earn money. Most teens her age are beginning to expand their social network of friends and begin dating. Many teens are often shy or nervous around the opposite sex, so these growing social circles help teens learn, and practice, necessary socialization skills. Group activities like sports or school clubs and programs are positive ways for teens to socialize.

Parties like the one Alyssa attended can be detrimental. The lack of adult supervision and presence can promote teens engaging in unsafe behavior like drinking alcohol. Most teens are naïve to alcohol and unaware of its effects or how many drinks are too many. Alyssa's inhibitions decreased from drinking, and she readily engaged in sexual activity that she might not otherwise have. Spontaneous sexual activity like Alyssa had with another teen often occurs without any contraception, thus increasing the potential for pregnancy or for STDs to occur. Alyssa would have been an ideal candidate for emergency contraception following the event (e.g., Plan B).

One sexual encounter can cause pregnancy for a teen. Alyssa did not believe she could be pregnant because of her history of irregular periods, so she ignored her missed period. Many teens like Alyssa fear telling their parents about what happened, and the relationship between the divorced parents did not promote open communication with their child. Alyssa was wise to discuss her situation with the school nurse; teachers, counselors, or other trusted adults could also be resources for teens.

Alyssa was able to identify the care she needed and was presented with options. These were choices with a significant impact to Alyssa's life, so having support from her family or social network could have been useful. Like many teens, Alyssa felt abortion was her best option when faced with the magnitude and consequence of being pregnant or having a baby. Abortion is a safe procedure with relatively low incidence of complications. Like most teen girls who undergo an abortion, Alyssa tolerated the procedure well with side effects. In the future, however, she is at risk for emotional feelings or regret that could surface at any time.

Health care practitioners address the need for contraception immediately and often offer various options that could work for a teen's lifestyle. Alyssa's experience with the situation is unique, and there is no way for her to predict if, of when, she would have sex again. Condoms are effective birth control only when they are used consistently and properly. If Alyssa's social life changes and she considers being sexually active again, she should explore options for birth control prior to engaging in sexual activity to prevent another unwanted pregnancy.

2. GINA KEEPS HER BABY BUT FACES MANY CHALLENGES

Gina is a 17-year-old Hispanic girl who has been in a monogamous relationship with her boyfriend, Juan, for over two years. Although they each continue to live at home with their own parents, Gina and Juan are able to see each other regularly at school but sneak out to find time alone for intimacy. They have been sexually active for most of their relationship, relying on condoms for birth control when they are available. Juan planned to join the military and then marry Gina as soon as his training was completed, having her move with him around the world on his various military deployments.

Gina's parents were not happy with Gina dating Juan. They did not like Juan and think he is a bad influence on their daughter. They disapprove of Gina and Juan's relationship and feel Juan is trying to steal their daughter away. They forbade Gina from seeing him and encouraged her to finish school.

Shortly after Juan left for the military, Gina discovered she was pregnant. Gina did not believe in abortion and knew she had to keep her baby. In addition, she knew Juan wanted her to keep the baby also and believed he would marry her in a few years once his military training was completed. Gina planned to live at home with her parents, continue to finish high school, and raise her baby until Juan returned.

Gina's parents were furious when she told them she was pregnant. Gina expected that her parents would be excited about the baby and the opportunity to become grandparents. Instead, Gina's parents voiced their disappointment, embarrassment, and anger that Gina got pregnant. They felt like they were betrayed and could no longer trust their daughter. If she insisted on raising the baby, she would have to do it on her own, including finding her own home. Gina's parents told her she had a few weeks to find a home and a way to support herself and the baby.

Gina shared what happened in her home with the midwife who was caring for her at the women's clinic. The midwife connected Gina with the clinic's social worker. The social worker listened to Gina's issues and realized Gina's living situation would not be ideal for Gina or her baby. The social worker explored all of Gina's options and tried to find viable solutions. In the end, the social worker helped secure Gina housing and enrolled her in various assistance programs so Gina could get food, items for the baby, basic utilities, and maintain her housing. Gina's parents continued to send her money when they could.

Gina tried to stay in school. Her high school has a program specifically designed for teen mothers who were pregnant to stay on track with their schoolwork. Unfortunately, Gina developed preeclampsia and was hospitalized for several weeks, delivering her baby early. Gina's baby spent 6 weeks in the neonatal intensive care unit before being discharged home to Gina.

Gina's baby had multiple needs once it was home, including continuous oxygen therapy and various medications to be administered throughout the day. Gina was unable to focus on her schoolwork and care for the baby at the same time. She skipped a year of school and hoped that when the baby was older, she could return and finish high school. Juan continued his military training and tried to send Gina money often. Gina's social worker provided support, encouragement, and access to additional resources.

Analysis

Teens form relationships that they believe will last for many years. Gina had strong feelings for Juan and believed that their relationship, and dreams or plans, would come to fruition. Teen girls who become pregnant often feel that having a baby is the next natural step in their relationship or that having a baby is a way to hold onto a boyfriend. In some cultures, having a baby while a partner is in the military is a way to preserve his legacy in the event he dies in the line of duty.

Parental disapproval of a boyfriend is common. However, measures at keeping the teens apart often fail, with teens sneaking out to meet each other. When parents dislike a teen girl's boyfriend, the lines of communication between the teen girl and her parents are broken and teens, therefore, will not feel comfortable speaking with their parents about critical situations like pregnancy.

Teen parents often feel a wide range of emotions when they learn their teen daughter is pregnant, including sadness, disappointment, embarrassment, and anger. Regardless of their feelings, and despite their dislike or disapproval of their daughter's boyfriend or situation, parents cannot kick their children out of their home and leave them homeless and without resources. The clinic midwife was correct to refer Gina to the social worker. Social workers are an invaluable resource for pregnant teens to secure housing and any additional resources a teen may need. Gina transitioned from the less ideal situation in her parents' home to her own home safely.

Teen mothers are susceptible to complications during pregnancy like gestational diabetes, preeclampsia, and premature birth. Women with preeclampsia may require prolonged hospitalization and monitoring; for teen mothers, this could mean missing a significant portion of school, thus delaying completion of a grade level. A premature baby also has significant needs, so Gina found herself unable to balance her schooling with managing the needs of a child.

Teen mothers can be great parents. Gina possessed the energy and determination to complete high school, raise her baby, and be with Juan. Many teen parents go on to have successful marriages, careers, and a family. Most teen parents, despite any adversity, remain hopeful and focused on a bright future and anticipate their dreams coming true.

3. MATT'S EXPERIENCE AS A TEEN FATHER

Matt, a high school senior, recently turned 18 and is planning to attend college on a sports scholarship in the fall. He has been dating 16-year-old Alexa for 6 months, and they have been sexually active since the beginning of their relationship. Matt tried to use condoms often but felt they were awkward to use and uncomfortable. Alexa told Matt that she had regular, predictable periods, and knew exactly when her fertile time was. Matt only changed to only using condoms during the times Alexa told him she might be fertile.

Alexa developed nausea, vomiting, abdominal discomfort, and fatigue. Believing she had a cold or the flu, Alexa ignored her symptoms for several days. However, when Alexa finally saw her health care practitioner, a pregnancy test was performed and confirmed that Alexa was about 8 weeks pregnant. Matt and Alexa have a decision to make: keep the baby, give it up for adoption, or for Alexa to have an abortion. Because of the couple's personal beliefs against abortion and their desire to raise their baby, Matt felt the only solution was to marry Alexa and raise the baby as a family.

Because Alexa was under 18 years of age, she could not freely marry Matt without parental consent. Although Alexa's parents were disappointed with the circumstances surrounding Alexa's pregnancy, they were happy that the couple opted to keep the baby and gave their permission for Alexa to marry Matt. Their parental consent was verified by two witnesses and approved by a judge when Matt and Alexa applied for a marriage license in their state.

The first months of their marriage were difficult. Matt completed high school but gave up his scholarship and plans for college. He found a job in a warehouse and worked as much overtime as he could to earn money. The couple was living with Alexa's parents while they saved money for their own home and to buy things for the baby. Alexa finished her junior year of high school but had to complete the final semester at home and take virtual classes after being diagnosed with preeclampsia and put on bed rest.

Around her 27th week of pregnancy Alexa developed sudden abdominal pain that came in frequent, unrelenting waves. As Matt rushed her to the hospital, Alexa started having heavy vaginal bleeding. On arrival to the hospital the delivery room team suspected Alexa was having a placental abruption and performed an emergency cesarean birth. The baby boy required resuscitation at birth and was extremely small for its gestational age.

The baby was in the neonatal ICU (NICU) for several months. During the first weeks in the NICU the baby had significant bleeding within the brain that caused permanent damage, thus contributing to severe developmental delay. The diagnosis meant the baby would need ongoing physical, occupational, and other supportive therapies well into his adulthood. The baby was also at risk for developing other complications during childhood.

Once the baby was discharged home, Matt and Alexa tried to raise the baby and provide for all its needs. A social worker helped the couple secure additional resources, but the medical bills for the baby continued to increase and surpassed what the couple was able to pay. It became a struggle for the couple to manage their own day-to-day expenses. Matt took on as much additional work as possible and was working various shifts at different jobs several days each week. The burden of caring for the baby fell mostly to Alexa. The couple argued frequently, and their relationship, and intimacy, deteriorated. The baby was never going to get better, and the couple knew their relationship was permanently damaged also.

Analysis

Matt and Alexa's situation is common. Teen couples share an intimate relationship, and their feelings intensify over time. Alexa was like many teen girls and believed her menstrual periods were regular enough to predict fertility. However, many teen girls have irregular ovulation despite consistent menstrual periods, making fertility unpredictable. Alexa's risk of pregnancy increased, thus the need for effective birth control. Pregnant teens are faced with several options, and many opt to marry to keep the baby. Some teens believe that they need to marry to legitimize the baby or their relationship, or to satisfy cultural, religious, or familial obligations. Many states in the United States, however, have stringent laws surrounding teen marriage and make the age of majority 18; teens under 18 years of age require parental permission and frequently a judge's approval to marry. Although some teen marriages are successful, most fail. Familial support and the availability of financial and other resources increases the likelihood of a teen marriage being sustained.

A teen pregnancy is susceptible to a host of complications. Alexa developed one of the most common complications found in teen mothers: preeclampsia. Preeclampsia is unpredictable and can quickly progress to other complications if not properly controlled. Even with proper treatment, however, complications like placental abruption can erupt quickly. The baby of a preeclamptic mother, like Mike and Alexa's, can be profoundly compromised because of these unforeseen complications. If the baby survives the birth, they are often susceptible to multiple complications after birth because of prematurity. Intraventricular hemorrhage, or severe bleeding within a baby's brain, is a common complication occurring in premature babies that can cause permanent, irreversible brain damage in babies like Matt and Alexa's.

A child with special needs can drain a family's resources; the child's needs for care and services only increase as the child ages. A couple, regardless of age, faces significant stressors that can compromise the integrity of their relationship. Research suggests that teen couples lack the stamina and perseverance to meet the challenges that a special needs child poses. Although some teen couples may be able to navigate the challenges of a special needs child, many do not unless significant resources, including social, familial, and financial, exist.

4. ERICA OPTS FOR ADOPTION

Erica is a 16-year-old high school junior. Erica attends her local public high school and is very popular among the students in her class. Although she is not a member of any clubs nor does she belong to any sports teams, Erica is familiar with many people in her school and within the towns surrounding her high school. Erica's reputation, however, preceded her. Erica became sexually active during her freshman year of high school, and she has had multiple sex partners since. To Erica, having sex while dating different boys is a sign of maturity. Boys dated Erica because they feel she was willing to have sex with anyone she dated.

By the time Erica reached her junior year of high school, she had already had several different sex partners. Erica relied on condoms as her most convenient form of birth control but admitted there were a few times where she had unprotected sex. Erica had never been pregnant before and felt she was both lucky to have avoided pregnancy and knowledgeable enough about her body to know when her fertile times were.

Erica realized she was pregnant when she had missed her period for over 2 weeks and had increasing hunger, breast tenderness, fatigue, and some nausea. She had taken a home pregnancy test that confirmed she was pregnant. Fortunately, Erica had a supportive mother and grandmother who helped her decide the best options for her. Erica knew she had to have this baby but knew she was in no position to raise a baby by herself. She was adamant that abortion was not an option. Erica knew she wanted to be part of her baby's life somehow but also acknowledged that another couple or parent would be in a better position to raise her baby.

Erica connected with a social worker referred to her by her health care practitioner's office. The social worker provided Erica with information about her options, including how the adoption process worked. Although Erica knew surrendering her baby for adoption would be difficult, she was comforted by the fact that she may have an opportunity to be part of her baby's life and that the baby would know who she is and have contact with her.

The social worker connected Erica with a lawyer who specialized in private adoption. To Erica's surprise there are many couples who wish to raise a baby while including the birth mother and her family in the baby's life. Erica answered many questions about her lifestyle, medical history, and background and as much of her family history that she knew. The lawyer took her information and promised to reconnect with her once a suitable family was found.

In a few weeks, the adoption lawyer contacted Erica with a potential family. This family was a young couple who desperately wanted a child but was unable to have their own baby. The adoption lawyer explained Erica's requests, and the potential adoptive parents were agreeable to the idea of an open adoption where Erica could continue to be a presence in the baby's life as its birth mother.

The adoption lawyer, Erica, and the prospective adoptive parents formalized an agreement. Erica would relinquish custody of the baby after it was born to the adoptive parents, but she would be identified as the birth mother. The adoptive family agreed to keep in regular contact with Erica throughout each year, including emails and photos of the baby, and Erica could see the baby several times throughout the year. Most important to Erica, the baby would know Erica was its mother, and Erica was allowed to be present at major milestones in the baby's life like birthdays or graduations. Further, Erica was allowed to contact the child by email, text, letters or in-person meetings throughout the child's life. Erica delivered a healthy baby girl, and the adoptive parents were present for the birth.

Erica, the adoptive parents, and the baby spent time together at the hospital after the delivery, and then the adoptive parents took the baby home. Erica was named as the birth mother on the birth certificate and was allowed regular visits with her daughter throughout the following years.

Analysis

Teenage girls often have multiple sex partners. Low self-esteem may lead teen girls toward sexual activity for validation of beauty or worth. The desire for attention, and the instant gratification of different sex partners, is alluring. Teenage girls who engage in various sex acts with different partners, however, often develop an unjustifiable reputation, especially among teenage boys, as "easy" or a girl one should have sex with. Although many teen girls are proactive in accessing birth control to prevent unwanted pregnancy, many teen girls do not have that option and rely on condoms or a perceived belief about their own menstrual cycles to determine fertility. Like Erica, many teen girls find their calculations of fertility are wrong and discover they are pregnant.

Erica is like many teen girls; they are opposed to abortion but realize they cannot raise a baby on their own. Wanting to provide the best for their baby, adoption is a logical consideration. However, modern teen mothers do not want to relinquish custody of their baby entirely; many teen mothers, and their families, want their baby to know who their mother is and be involved in their baby's life. Thus, the shame and secrecy surrounding a baby born out of wedlock of prior decades has disappeared.

There are many attorneys who work with families to secure an adoption agreed on by the birth mother and the adopting couple with the influence of an intermediary like social services or child welfare agencies. These private adoptions allow the birth mother and the adoptive family the freedom to customize the adoption agreement. Although Erica's adoption conditions and agreement are unique, there was significant latitude to negotiate an agreement that would work for both Erica and the adoptive parents. Erica's baby was adopted by a loving, nurturing family that recognized the role Erica played in the child's life.

5. MARYANNE HAS A COMPLICATED AND DIFFICULT PREGNANCY

Maryanne is a 14-year-old high school freshman who began dating a boy she met in one of her classes. Maryanne had become sexually active in the seventh grade and had engaged in sexual activity with every boy she dated. Maryanne was happy: she enjoyed high school, had lots of friends, and she had a boyfriend. However, Maryanne's world changed when she found out she was unexpectedly pregnant.

Maryanne experienced the symptoms of pregnancy very early. She had persistent headaches, was always feeling nauseous, and had no appetite. Her breasts were tender and painful, and wearing a bra or tight clothing caused her more discomfort. When her period was late, she took a home pregnancy test that confirmed she was pregnant. Maryanne was nervous and concerned about being pregnant; the more she worried about the future, the worse her symptoms seemed to be. She knew she needed help from someone she trusted. Maryanne shared the news about her pregnancy with her older sister and, with her sister's help, secured an appointment with a health care practitioner. After the initial examination and testing was complete, the health care practitioner discussed Maryanne's options about having the baby and described what Maryanne could expect over the next weeks of pregnancy. Later, Maryanne and her sister told their parents together about Maryanne's pregnancy. The family made the decision together that Maryanne would keep the baby, and the family would help her raise it. The father of the baby's family also agreed to support Maryanne and the baby.

Maryanne was relieved to have her family's support. However, her physical symptoms did not go away. The health care practitioner reassured Maryanne that her symptoms would likely improve by the second trimester; Maryanne continued to feel worse. Because she was becoming weaker, could not eat sufficient food to gain weight, and had frequent vomiting, Maryanne required hospitalization to provide her intravenous medications and fluids to alleviate her symptoms. Maryanne improved slightly but was unable to return to school.

Maryanne's symptoms persisted. She continued to lose weight and was malnourished. Her health care practitioner coordinated home infusion services where nurses came to Maryanne's home and administered continuous intravenous nutrition that infused over 24-hour periods. The health care practitioner became concerned that Maryanne's baby was not growing properly and was falling behind on its expected growth. Maryanne's blood pressure began to increase, and she developed lingering, often severe, headaches. Maryanne was readmitted to the hospital around 28 weeks gestation and was going to stay there until she delivered.

Maryanne became more depressed and anxious. She was scared to be in the hospital and nervous about what would happen to the baby. She felt isolated from all her friends and was concerned about falling too far behind in school. She began losing sleep and was feeling increasingly frustrated and irritable. Social workers and the nurses in the hospital tried to offer her support and diversionary activities.

Maryanne's baby continued to grow poorly, and her persistent high blood pressures began to impact the blood flow to the placenta. A decision was made to induce Maryanne's labor. The induction went well, but Maryanne's labor did not progress as expected because the baby would not descend properly, raising fears that the baby might be too large for Maryanne's small pelvis. As the delivery room team tried to increase the strength of Maryanne's contractions, the baby began to show signs that it could not tolerate labor. As the baby's heart rate continued to drop, another decision was made to perform a cesarean birth. A baby girl was delivered that went immediately to the neonatal intensive care unit (NICU).

Maryanne was able to go home within 4 days, but her baby would require several weeks of care in the NICU. Maryanne remained weak, had persistent pain, and needed help to get to the bathroom or bathe. Visiting her daughter in the NICU was particularly tiring for her, and she was unable to produce sufficient breast milk to breastfeed her baby, so the baby needed to be supplemented with formula. Maryanne's incision line became infected, and she was admitted to the hospital again for antibiotic therapy. She continued to lose weight and became more depressed about her inability to care for herself or her baby. Although the health care practitioner reassured Maryanne that she would heal, she still had several months ahead of her to fully recover and resume her usual activities.

Analysis

Teens are having their first sexual encounters, including sexual intercourse, as early as junior high or grammar school in the United States. There is a belief, perhaps popularized by social media, television, or the movies that dating, relationships, and intimacy signify maturity, worthiness, acceptance, or popularity. Teens who have sex at younger ages, like Maryanne, often lack access to a proper and consistent form of birth control and are highly susceptible to pregnancy.

Women experience symptoms of pregnancy differently. However, pregnant teens often have more pronounced and persistent symptoms that can be debilitating. Prolonged vomiting and lack of sufficient intake of nutrients can quickly lead to malnutrition for mothers. The baby can also display the effects of poor nutrition with delayed growth. Mothers like Maryanne often require hospitalization and, if conventional treatments are unsuccessful, may need ongoing intravenous therapy to provide nutrition either in the hospital or in the home. Despite treatment, babies can continue to fall behind in expected growth when mothers are undernourished.

Preeclampsia, common in teen mothers like Maryanne, can also complicate a baby's growth. Prolonged and poorly controlled high blood pressure causes damage to the placenta and its vascular bed that can continue to impede a baby's growth. Babies of preeclamptic, malnourished mothers often require imminent delivery despite being premature or small because the risk of intrauterine fetal death is too high. Mothers who need to deliver their babies will have their labor induced with medication. However, babies like Maryanne's may not properly enter the pelvis or tolerate the increasing intensity of labor, so a cesarean birth is often the only safe route of delivery.

A cesarean birth can have complications. Although most mothers tolerate the procedure well and heal quickly, mothers like Maryanne who had complications during pregnancy recover slower. Infections of the incision line can occur that further delay healing. The complications during pregnancy and surrounding the delivery of the baby take their toll on women, especially teen mothers like Maryanne. Maryanne was susceptible to depression, confusion, frustration, anger, worthlessness, or feeling overwhelmed and anxious. Teens may face a prolonged recovery that can interfere with bonding with the baby, thus increasing the various emotions a teen mother may face.

Family support is essential. Maryanne was fortunate to have parents, an older sibling, and involvement with the father of the baby's family to support her. A teen's future plans can change, but families provide encouragement and assistance to meet future challenges and navigate any obstacles a new mother, or a new family, may face.

Glossary

Abandonment: A parent's choice to willfully withhold physical, emotional, and financial support from a minor child.

Abortion: The ending, or termination, of a pregnancy.

Adoption: Giving someone else the legal right and responsibility to raise your child.

Age of majority: The age at which a person is granted by law the rights (e.g., ability to sue) and responsibilities (e.g., liability under contract) of an adult.

Amenorrhea: The absence of a menstrual period or a missed period.

Amniocentesis: A sampling of amniotic fluid using a hollow needle inserted into the uterus during pregnancy.

Amniotic fluid: The fluid surrounding a fetus inside the uterus during pregnancy.

Anemia: A condition marked by a deficiency of red blood cells or of hemoglobin in the blood.

Apgar score: A score assigned after birth at 1 and 5 minutes of life, and checks a baby's heart rate, muscle tone, and other signs to determine if extra medical care or emergency care is needed.

Areola: A small circular area, in particular the ring of pigmented skin surrounding a nipple.

Attention-deficit/hyperactivity disorder (ADHD): A chronic condition including attention difficulty, hyperactivity, and impulsiveness.

Baby Blues: Temporary symptoms of depression affecting a woman within 1 to 2 weeks after giving birth.

Bilirubin: An orange-yellow pigment formed in the liver by the breakdown of hemoglobin and excreted in bile.

Bloody show: A type of vaginal discharge that contains mucus tinged with either bright red or dark brown blood. It occurs during the end of a pregnancy, just before a woman goes into labor.

Bonding: The attachment that forms between an infant and its mother beginning at birth. Maternal-infant bonding influences the child's psychological and physical development.

Braxton Hicks contractions: Painless uterine contractions beginning around week 12 and occurring throughout the pregnancy. These contractions typically cease with walking or other forms of exercise. Unlike uterine contractions associated with labor, Braxton Hicks do not cause the cervix to dilate.

Breech: Presentation of a baby in which the face, buttocks, legs, or feet are nearest the cervix and emerge first at birth.

Cephalopelvic disproportion: Occurs when a baby's head or body is too large to fit through the mother's pelvis.

Cerebral palsy: A group of disorders that affect a person's ability to move and maintain balance and posture due to brain injury or damage during pregnancy or delivery.

Chorionic villi: Microscopic, finger-like projections inside the uterus that contain capillaries for blood to flow through to allow the transfer of nutrients from the mother's blood to the fetus.

Chorionic villi sampling: A test made in early pregnancy to detect congenital abnormalities in the fetus. A tiny tissue sample is taken from the villi of the chorion, which forms the fetal part of the placenta.

Civic responsibility: The duties of all citizens to take an active role in society and to consider the interests and concerns of other individuals in the community.

Closed adoption: An adoption where no identifying information about the birth family or the adoptive family is shared between the two, and there is no contact between the two families.

Colostrum: A sticky white or yellow fluid secreted by the breasts during the second half of pregnancy and for a few days after birth, before breast milk comes in.

Community college: Two-year public institutions that grant certificates, diplomas, or associate degrees.

Conception: Also called fertilization, the act of the sperm cell traveling up the vagina to unite with the egg in the fallopian tube.

Cooperative education: A structured method of combining classroom-based education with practical work experience.

Cord prolapse: An obstetrical emergency where the umbilical cord slips down into the birth canal, leading to decreased circulation to the baby.

Decelerations: Sudden or prolonged drops in the baby's heart rate.

Deoxyribonucleic acid (DNA): The molecule that contains the genetic code of organisms.

DNA paternity testing: The use of DNA profiles to determine whether an individual is the biological parent of another individual.

Dyslexia: A learning disorder that involves difficulty reading due to problems identifying speech sounds and learning how they relate to letters and words.

Ectopic pregnancy: A pregnancy that has implanted outside the uterus.

Effacement: The process by which the cervix prepares for delivery. After the baby has engaged in the pelvis, it gradually drops closer to the cervix. The cervix will gradually soften, shorten, and become thinner.

Emancipation: When an individual has reached the age of majority under applicable law and has the right to become independent of his or her parents' control.

Endometriosis: A condition resulting from the appearance of endometrial tissue outside the uterus and causing adhesions and pelvic pain.

Endometrium: The mucous membrane lining the uterus, which thickens during the menstrual cycle in preparation for possible implantation of an embryo.

Epidural anesthesia: Regional anesthesia that blocks nerve impulses from the lower spinal segments to relieve pain in a particular region of the body.

Episiotomy: A surgical cut made at the opening of the vagina during childbirth, to aid a difficult delivery and prevent rupture of tissues.

Fertilization: When a sperm and egg unite after ovulation.

Gestation: The process of carrying, or being carried within, the womb between conception and birth.

Gestational diabetes: A condition characterized by an elevated level of glucose in the blood during pregnancy, typically resolving after the birth.

Graduate Education Development (GED) test: An educational test to determine whether a person has achieved a high school–level education.

Hegar's sign: The softening of the uterine cervix and lower uterine segment palpated during a pelvic examination.

Hemorrhage: Heavy, persistent, and uncontrolled bleeding.

High blood pressure: A common condition in which the long-term force of the blood against your artery walls is high enough that it may eventually cause health problems, such as heart disease.

Hormones: Regulatory substances produced in an organism and transported in tissue fluids such as blood or to stimulate specific cells or tissues into action.

Human chorionic gonadotropin (HCG): The pregnancy hormone whose levels rise then predictably fall during the early weeks of pregnancy.

Hydatidiform mole: An abnormal growth of a fertilized egg.

Hydrocephalus: The buildup of fluid in the cavities or ventricles deep within the brain. The excess fluid increases the size of the ventricles and puts pressure on the brain.

Hyperactivity: Behavior that is usually constant activity, being easily distracted, impulsiveness, inability to concentrate, aggressiveness, and similar behaviors.

Incest: Sexual activity between family members or close relatives.

Intraventricular hemorrhage: Bleeding into the fluid-filled areas, or ventricles, inside the brain. The condition occurs most often in babies that are born early or premature.

Jaundice: The yellowing of the skin caused by increased levels of bilirubin.

Joint custody: Both parents of a child share major decision making regarding, for example, education, medical care, and religious upbringing, and the child spends equal or close to equal amount of time with both parents.

Lactation: The secretion of milk by the mammary glands.

Lactiferous ducts: Ducts that converge and form a branched system connecting the nipple to the lobules of the mammary gland. When breast milk is produced, under the influence of hormones, the milk is moved to the nipple by the action of smooth muscle contractions along the ductal system to the tip of the nipple.

Legal custody: The right awarded to the parents to make important decisions regarding the child's life.

Let-down reflex: Stimulation of the nerves in the breast through the action of an infant suckling at the breast to release the milk from the milk ducts.

Lightening: A drop in the level of the uterus during the last weeks of pregnancy as the head of the fetus engages in the pelvis.

Mammary glands: Glands located in the breasts of females that are responsible for the production of breast milk.

Mandated reporter: People who have regular contact with vulnerable people and are therefore legally required to ensure a report is made when abuse is observed or suspected.

Matrimony: The state or ceremony of being married.

Medicaid: In the United States is a federal and state program that helps with medical costs for some people with limited income and resources.

Menstruation: A woman's monthly period, or the predictable days of vaginal bleeding that occur about the same time each month.

Miscarriage: Loss or end of a pregnancy prior to birth.

Montgomery tubercles: Sebaceous (oil) glands that appear as small bumps around the dark area of the nipple. Their primary function is lubricating and keeping germs away from the breasts.

Mucus plug: A thick clump of cervical mucus that forms during pregnancy, helping block the cervix.

Nesting: During pregnancy is the overwhelming desire to get the home ready for a new baby. The nesting instinct is strongest in the later weeks coming upon delivery.

Open adoption: Allows for some form of contact or association between the birth parents, the adoptive parents, and the adopted child.

Order of Filiation: A court order that names a man as the father of a child. An Order of Filiation gives the father the right to custody of the child, the right to visitation with the child, and the responsibility of paying child support.

Ovulation: When an egg is released from an ovary during the menstrual cycle.

Parenthood: Carrying a baby until it is born, or completing a pregnancy, and raising the child. Also, adopting and raising a child.

Paternity: The state of being someone's father.

Pelvic inflammatory disease: Inflammation of the female genital tract, accompanied by fever and lower abdominal pain, commonly caused by untreated or persistent sexually transmitted infections.

Perinatal asphyxia: A condition that describes decreased levels of oxygen to the baby during labor or the childbirth process.

Perineum: The skin and tissues between the vaginal opening and the anus.

Physical custody: A parent's right to have the child to reside with him or her.

Placental abruption: Occurs when the placenta separates from the inner wall of the uterus before birth.

Postpartum depression (PPD): Depression suffered by a mother following childbirth, typically arising from the combination of hormonal changes, psychological adjustment to motherhood, and fatigue.

Post-traumatic stress disorder (PTSD): A mental health condition that is triggered by a terrifying event either by experiencing it or witnessing it. Symptoms may include flashbacks, nightmares, and severe anxiety, as well as uncontrollable thoughts about the event.

Preeclampsia: A pregnancy complication characterized by high blood pressure and signs of damage to another organ system, most often the liver and kidneys. Preeclampsia usually begins after 20 weeks of pregnancy in women whose blood pressure had been normal.

Pregnancy-induced hypertension: The development of new hypertension in a pregnant woman after 20 weeks' gestation without the presence of protein in the urine or other signs of preeclampsia.

Premature labor: The onset of labor prior to 37 weeks gestation.

Prolactin: The hormone that makes breast milk when a woman is pregnant or breastfeeding.

Rape: A type of sexual violence with forced or alcohol/drug-facilitated anal, oral, or vaginal penetration.

Rape-related pregnancy (RRP): Pregnancy that a rape victim attributes to rape.

Relaxin: A hormone secreted by the placenta that causes the cervix to dilate and prepares the uterus for the action of oxytocin during labor.

Reproductive coercion: A form of sexual violence that involves exerting power or control over reproduction through interference with contraception use and pregnancy pressure.

Safe Haven: Statutes that vary by that which allow parents of any age to leave an unharmed newborn at designated safe places like hospitals, police stations, or fire stations without the fear of criminal charges for abandonment.

Sexual debut: The age when a person has their first experience of sexual intercourse.

Shoulder dystocia: A birth injury that happens when one or both of a baby's shoulders get stuck inside the mother's pelvis during labor.

Sole custody: A specific type of child custody arrangement in which only one parent or legal guardian is granted both physical and legal custody of the child.

Sonogram: A noninvasive diagnostic test that uses sound waves to explore the uterus to identify, and confirm, the presence of a fetus.

Statutory rape: Nonforcible sexual activity in which one of the individuals is below the age of consent.

Striae gravidarum: The presence of dark streaking to the skin of the abdomen.

Telehealth: The distribution of health-related services and information via electronic information and telecommunication technologies (like telephones or computers).

Transition: The final phase of the first stage of labor where the cervix dilates from 7 to 10 centimeters.

Truancy: Any intentional, unjustified, unauthorized, or illegal absence from compulsory education. It is a deliberate absence by a student's own free will and usually does not refer to legitimate excused absences, such as ones related to medical conditions.

Uterine ballottement: When the lower uterine segment or cervix is tapped by a health care practitioner's fingers during a pelvic examination, the sensation of the fetus floating upward then sinking backward is felt.

Vocational school: A type of school designed to provide technical skills required to complete tasks of a particular, and specific, job.

Directory of Resources

BOOKS

Frohnapfel-Krueger, L. (2010). *Teen pregnancy and parenting*. Farmington Hills, MI: Greenhaven Publishing.

Murkoff, H. (2016). *What to expect when you're expecting*. 5th ed. New York: Workman Publishing.

Quinn, P. (2018). *Sexually transmitted diseases: Your questions answered*. Santa Barbara, CA: ABC-CLIO/Greenwood.

Quinn, P. (2019). *Birth control: Your questions answered*. Santa Barbara, CA: ABC-CLIO/Greenwood.

Rezvani, F. (2020). *The perfect living womb. Conversations with my virtual pregnant patient: A concise, informative guide to pregnancy and beyond from an OB/GYN*. Printed by author.

HOTLINES

Boys Town National Hotline—a free resource and counseling service that assists youth (male and female) and parents 24/7, year-round, nationwide. **(800)448-3000.**

Covenant House Nine Line—a free, confidential crisis hotline for youth and parents that provides information about shelters, health services, and crisis intervention. **(800)999-9999.**

National Runaway Switchboard—a national communications system that assists youth who have run away or are considering running away and their families. **(800)RUNAWAY/(800)786-2929.**

National Sexual Assault Hotline—a free, confidential service that provides support and connects victims of sexual assault (male and female) with resources within their community. **(800)656-HOPE.**

WEBSITES

American Association of Blood Banks—the leading accrediting institution that certifies laboratories for paternity testing and provides resources for finding local accredited laboratories for DNA paternity testing.

DNA Paternity Testing Facilities
http://www.aabb.org/sa/facilities/Pages/RTestAccrFac.aspx

American Pregnancy Association—a national health organization committed to promoting reproductive and pregnancy wellness through education, support, advocacy, and community awareness.

Pregnant Teen
https://americanpregnancy.org/unplanned-pregnancy/pregnant-teen

American Sexual Health Association—promotes the sexual health of individuals, families, and communities to foster healthy sexual behaviors and relationships and prevent adverse health outcomes.
http://www.ashasexualhealth.org

Centers for Disease Control and Prevention (CDC)—an agency that works to protect the nation from health, safety, and security threats, both in the United States and foreign. The CDC connects both state and local health departments across the country to discover patterns of disease, provide statistics, and respond or provide resources when needed.

Rape-Related Pregnancy
https://www.cdc.gov/violenceprevention/datasources/nisvs/understanding-RRP-inUS.html

Teen Pregnancy
www.cdc.org/teenpregnancy/about/index.htm

Vaccines for Children Schedule
www.cdc.gov/vaccines/parents/by-age/birth.html

Child Welfare—a government agency that provides access to information and resources to help protect children and strengthen families, including information about child abuse, child welfare, and adoption. www.childwelfare.gov

Children by Choice—an international organization that provides unbiased information on all unplanned pregnancy options including abortion, adoption, and parenting. www.childrenbychoice.org.au

Do Something—a global nonprofit organization with the goal of motivating young people to make positive changes both online and offline through campaigns that make an impact. www.dosomething.org

Graduate Education Development (GED) test—the official online resource to prepare for and earn a high school equivalency diploma. www.GED.com

Guttmacher Institute—an organization that studies reproductive health policy.

U.S. Laws by State Regarding Abortion
https://www.guttmacher.org/state-policy/explore/overview-abortion-laws

Hague Convention—an international agreement to safeguard intercountry adoptions and provides current regulations when considering international adoption.
https://travel.state.gov/content/travel/en/Intercountry-Adoption /Adoption-Process/understanding-the-hague-convention.html

Healthy Teen Network—an organization that provides adolescents and young adults—including young people who are pregnant or parenting—comprehensive, confidential support, information, and services, including contraceptive services, and if pregnant, to full options counseling and services.
www.healthyteennetwork.org

Medical Institute for Sexual Health—an online resource for medically accurate, up-to-date information about sexual health. www.medinstitute.org

National Abortion Federation (NAF)—an organization of abortion providers who provide information about abortion and funding assistance. www.prochoice.org

National Association of Social Workers—the website for the National Association of Social Workers that provides information on various physical and mental health related topics and a link to find a social worker. www.helpstartshere.org

National Runaway Safeline—a national communication system for runaway or homeless youth that provides services, information, and education for youth, parents, and communities. www.1800runaway.org

Parentology.com—a website dedicated to providing current news, trends, or other information about all aspects of parenting. www.parentology.com

U.S. Department of Health and Human Services, Child Welfare Information Gateway—Supporting Pregnant & Parenting Teens—links to various information on parenting tips and state and local resources to support pregnant and parenting teens. https://www.childwelfare.gov/topics/preventing/promoting/parenting /pregnant-teens

Verywell Family—Verywell Family is a modern resource that offers a realistic and friendly approach to pregnancy and parenting. https://www.verywellfamily.com

Women Deserve Better—A compilation of practical resources and inspirational stories from women and men who have faced challenges regarding pregnancy at work, home, life, school, and relationships. www.womendeservebetter.com

World Health Organization—a specialized agency of the United Nations responsible for international public health; they provide statistics, information, and resources about health issues from an international perspective.

Teen Pregnancy Statistics
www.who.int/news-room/fact-sheets/detail/adolescent-pregnancy

Adoption

Adoption for My Baby—a website that provides women with a variety of information about adoption and assists to connect them with qualified adoption specialists. www.adoption-for-my-baby.com

Adoption Exchange—a nonprofit organization that that provides pre- and postadoption services that help waiting children in foster care get established in permanent homes.
www.adoptex.org

American Adoptions—a nonprofit national adoption agency that provides useful information about adoption.
www.americanadoptions.com

Sexual Assault

Futures without Violence—an organization that provides resources to empower individuals and organizations working to end violence against women and children around the world.
www.futureswithoutviolence.org

Love Is Respect—an organization dedicated to engage, educate, and empower young people to prevent and end abusive relationships.
www.loveisrespect.org

National Center on Domestic and Sexual Violence—an agency that offers consulting, training, and advocacy on issues relating to domestic violence and sexual abuse.
www.ncdsv.org

National Center on Violence and Sexual Assault Prevention—based out of the University of Michigan, they offer resources to eradicate sexual assault, stalking, sexual harassment, and intimate partner violence.
http://m.sapac.umich.edu

National Sexual Violence Resource Center—the National Sexual Violence Resource Center is the leading nonprofit in providing information and tools to prevent and respond to sexual violence.
www.nsvrc.org

911Rape—this site offers support for sexual assault victims as well as a safe, anonymous way to learn how to get help after a sexual assault.
www.911rape.org

Project Respect—an international organization that brings together youth and adults to work to create awareness and dialogue around sexualized violence.
www.yesmeansyes.com

Rape, Abuse & Incest National Network (RAINN)—the nation's largest anti-sexual violence organization, RAINN created and operates the National Sexual Assault Hotline (800-656-HOPE) and partners local sexual assault service providers across the country. They also provide programs to prevent sexual violence, help victims, and ensure that perpetrators are brought to justice.
www.rainn.org

Teen Employment

U.S. Department of Labor—provides links to each state's labor laws and child labor laws.
https://www.dol.gov/agencies/whd/state

U.S Department of Labor Programs & Services—a guide to local and regional U.S. Department of Labor services (e.g., Workman's Compensation, apprenticeships, minimum wage requirements).
https://www.dol.gov/general/location

Youth Rules!—a website with links to resources that provides information regarding youth employment.
www.youthrules.gov

Index

Abandonment, 41–42, 101–102;
child, 42
Abortion: case study, 111–113;
complications, 30–32;
confidentiality and, 32; costs,
27–30; decisions about, 21;
induction, 27; infant, 36; informed
decision-making, 33; international,
36; Internet information and,
22; medical, 20–25; parental
permission and, 32; privacy rights
and, 22; regret and, 32; resources
for information, 33; state laws
and, 32–33; vacuum aspiration,
25–26
Additional Child Tax Credit, 40
Agency adoption, 36. See also
Adoption
Adoption, 33–37, 42; case study,
118–120; foster care and, 35; open,
35; private, 36; process for, 34–35;
through identification, 36; types of,
35–37

Affordable Care Act, 52. See also
Health insurance
Age of majority, 78, 80. See also Legal
concerns
Apgar score, 64–65

Baby Blues, 73
Baby Bump, 96
Barrier methods, 68–69; condoms, 69;
diaphragm, 68. See also Birth control
Biological father, 94. See also Teen
fathers
Birth, 56–58; baby needs after, 64–66;
cervical dilatation and, 56–58;
cesarean, 59–61; complications for
teens, 61–63; vaginal, 58–59
Birth control, 69–70; barrier methods,
68–69; condoms, 69; diaphragm,
68. See also Contraception
Birth rates, 3; geographic differences
and, 3; Hispanic teens and, 3;
non-Hispanic black teens and, 3;
non-Hispanic white teens and, 3

Bloody show, 55. *See also* Labor
Braxton Hicks contractions, 46, 49,
    53–55. *See also* Pregnancy
Breastfeeding, 66–68; benefits
    of, 66–67; let-down reflex, 68;
    prolactin, 68
Bullying, 6; sensitivity and, 6

Case studies, 111–123; abortion,
    111–113; adoption, 118–120;
    complications during pregnancy,
    120–123; teen father, 116–118;
    teen parents, 114–116
Cephalopelvic disproportion (CPD),
    61
Cervical dilatation, 56–58. *See also*
    Birth
Cesarean birth, 59; indications for,
    60–61. *See also* Birth
Child Care Assistance Program, 41
Child Health Insurance Plan
    (CHIP), 39, 52
Child Only health plans, 53
Child Protective Services (CPS), 91;
    removal of a child and, 91
Child Tax Credit, 40
Children, 10; long-term effects and
    teen pregnancy, 10–11
Closed adoption, 35. *See also*
    Adoption
College, 108–110; community,
    109; cooperative education,
    109; universities and, 109–110;
    vocational schools and, 109
Community resources, 19; health
    care services and, 19
Complications and pregnancy, 61–63
Conception, 44, 49, 93–94. *See also*
    Menstrual cycle
Condoms, 69. *See also* Barrier
    methods; Birth control;
    Contraception
Contraception, 5, 68–70; attitudes
    toward, 5; barrier methods, 68–69;

hormonal, 69; intrauterine device,
    70; long acting, 70; options for, 5
Culture, 8; teen pregnancy and, 8
Custody, 83–84; joint, 84; legal, 84;
    physical, 84; sole, 84; teen fathers
    and, 83–84

Dating, 6; parental involvement
    and, 18
Definitive signs of pregnancy, 46
Depo-Provera, 70. *See also* Progestin
Depression, 48. *See also* Pregnancy
Diaphragm, 68. *See also* Barrier
    methods; Birth control
Dilatation and evacuation, 26.
    See also Surgical abortion
DNA paternity testing, 82, 94–96;
    amniocentesis and, 95; chorionic
    villi sampling (CVS) and, 95;
    non-invasive prenatal paternity
    (NIPP) testing and, 95
Domestic violence, 98; pregnancy
    and, 98–99
Drug and alcohol use, 5; risk factors
    in teen pregnancy, 5

Earned Income Tax Credit, 40
Economic factors and pregnancy, 12;
    family and, 12
Ectopic pregnancy, 24
Education: societal risk factors and, 7;
    targeted, 18–19
Emancipation, 78–79. *See also* Legal
    concerns
Emergency Food Assistance Program,
    40
Emotional factors and pregnancy, 12;
    family and, 12
Employment, 103–105; exceptions
    for teens, 104; Fair Labor
    Standards Act and, 104; jobs for
    teens, 105; laws and, 103–104
Estrogen, 44, 67, 69, 71. *See also*
    Menstrual cycle

Fair Labor Standards Act, 104
Fertility, 70–72
Financial resources, 7, 40; assistance for mothers and children, 40–41; lack of and teen pregnancy, 7; non-profit organizations and, 41
First trimester, 48–49
Foster care, 35. *See also* Adoption

General education development/ graduate equivalency diploma (GED), 39, 107
Group B strep, 49–50

Head Start programs, 41
Health care policy, and abortion, 30
Health insurance, 52–53; parental coverage and, 52
Hegar's sign, 45
High school, 105–108; child care and, 107
Home Energy Assistance Program, 41
Homelessness, 102–103
Homeschooling, 103, 106; virtual programs and, 107
Housing, 101–103; alternatives for, 102; "kicked out," 102; parents and, 101–102. *See also* Parental involvement
Housing Choice Program, 41
Human chorionic gonadotropin (HCG), 46

Incest, 87; abortion and, 88; laws and, 88; long-term consequences of, 88–89; pregnancy and, 88; PTSD and, 89; punishment for, 88; rape and, 88
Induction abortion, 27; complications of, 27; procedure for, 27; recovery after, 27
Infant adoption, 36. *See also* Adoption

Infant needs, 37–38; costs and, 37
Insurance coverage, 29; teen parents and, 79
International adoption, 36. *See also* Adoption
Intrauterine device (IUD), 70

Joint custody, 84. *See also* Custody

Labor, 53, 56; active, 57; failure of, 61; relaxin, 54; stages of, 56–59; transition, 57; uterine contractions and, 53–55
Legal concerns, 75–91; DNA paternity testing and, 82; emancipation, 78–79; financial support for teen parents, 79; for grandchildren, 78; insurance coverage, 79; marriage, 80–81; neglect and, 79; parental involvement, 75; parental notification, 75; parental responsibilities for pregnant teen, 77; parents of teen father and, 80; removal of teen from the home, 77, 79; teen father and, 79–80, 81–83; teen living at home and, 76; teen mother rights, 78
Legal custody, 84. *See also* Custody
Legal guardian, 79
Let-down reflex, 68. *See also* Breastfeeding
Lightening, 54
Low birth weight, 64
Luteinizing hormone, 44

Mandated reporters, 90–91
Marriage, 80–81; laws and, 80; parental consent and, 80; teens and, 80
Media, 13; negative influence and, 16; positive influence of, 16; teen pregnancy and, 14
Medicaid, 39, 52

Medical abortion, 20–25;
    complications of, 30;
    contraindications for, 24;
    medications for, 24; side effects of,
    24. *See also* Abortion
Menstrual cycle, 43–44; calculating
    fertility and, 93–94; estrogen and,
    67, 71; ovulation, 44
Mental health, 72–73; after delivery,
    73; postpartum depression and,
    73; stress and, 72; teen pregnancy
    and, 72
Mifepristone, 24
Mini pill, 69–70. *See also* Progestin
Misoprostol, 24

National School Lunch Program, 40
Neglect, 79. *See also* Legal concerns
Neighborhoods, 7; impact of, 7;
    segregation and, 8
Newborn illnesses and emergencies,
    66
Newborn screening tests, 65

Open adoption, 35. *See also*
    Adoption
Order of Filiation, 83, 94
Ovulation, 44. *See also* Menstrual
    cycle

Parental involvement: child care
    and, 77; communication and, 17;
    dating and, 18; decisions regarding
    pregnancy, 76; expectations for,
    77–78; feelings and, 76; housing
    and, 101–103; obligations for,
    101–102; pregnancy prevention
    and, 17; role modeling, 77; support
    and, 75, 101–102
Paternity, 94. *See also* DNA paternity
    testing
Pell grants, 40
Physical custody, 84. *See also* Custody
Placenta, 58, 62

Polycystic ovarian syndrome
    (PCOS), 71
Postpartum depression, 73–74.
    See also Mental health
Post-traumatic stress disorder
    (PTSD), 73; incest and, 89; rape
    and, 86
Poverty, 6, 7, 11; children and, 11;
    society and, 7
Pre-eclampsia, 9, 47
Pregnancy, 9, 44–46; Baby Bump, 96;
    clothing for, 97; college and, 108;
    complications and, 9; concealing,
    97; dating and, 99–100; depression
    and, 48; friendships and, 100–101;
    high school and, 103–104,
    105–107; relationships and,
    98–99; showing, 96–97; signs and
    symptoms of, 44–45; social life
    and, 100–101; trimesters, 48–50
Pregnancy-induced hypertension
    (PIH), 9, 47
Premature birth, 47
Premature labor, 53
Prematurity, 9, 11; low birth weight
    and, 11
Prenatal care, 49, 50–52
Presumptive signs of pregnancy,
    44–45
Private adoption, 36. *See also*
    Adoption
Probable signs of pregnancy, 45–46
Progesterone, 67–68
Progestin, 69; Depo Provera and, 70.
    See also Mini pill
Prolactin, 68. *See also* Breastfeeding

Rape, 85–87; medical care after, 86;
    national hotline, 83; pregnancy
    and, 87; prosecution of, 86–87;
    PTSD and, 86; reporting, 86
Rape-Related Pregnancy (RRP), 87.
    See also Rape
Relaxin, 54. *See also* Labor

Residential programs, 106–107
Resources for child care, 38–40
Risk factors for teen pregnancy,
  4–7; family, 6; individual, 5–6;
  social, 6
Romeo and Juliet laws, 89–90.
  See also Statutory rape
Runaways, 102; national runaway
  switchboard, 102

Safe Haven statutes, 41
School performance, 5; drop out, 104;
  quitting and, 103; teen pregnancy
  and, 5; truancy, 103
Sex: consensual and teens, 89; minors
  and, 89; statutory rape and, 89
Sex abuse, 5
Sexual activity, 5
Sexually transmitted diseases (STDs),
  8, 47; fertility and, 71; teen
  mothers and, 8
16 & Pregnant, 15–16
Social factors, 12; family and, 12
Social worker, 38, 42, 52, 74, 76–77,
  79, 83, 85–86, 103
Societal factors, 7–8; teen pregnancy
  and, 7–8
Sole custody, 84. *See also* Custody
Stages of labor, 56–59. *See also* Labor
Statutory rape, 89; laws and, 89;
  prosecution of, 90. *See also* Romeo
  and Juliet laws
Sterilization, 70
Stress: child care and, 41; mental
  health and, 72–73
Striae gravidarum, 46
Supplemental Nutrition Assistance
  Program (SNAP), 39
Surgical abortion, 22, 26–27;
  complications, 26, 31–32; follow-up
  care, 26; procedure for, 26

Teen fathers, 9–10, 79–85; adoption
  and, 82–83; custody and visitation,

82; "deadbeat dad," 9; marriage
  and, 81; paternity confirmation,
  81–82; responsibility for teen
  mother, 79–80; rights and
  responsibilities of, 81–83; stigma
  and, 9; unborn baby and, 82;
  work and, 9
Teen Mom, 15
Teen mothers, 8–9; plan for
  pregnancy, 78
Teen parents, 8–10
Teen pregnancy, 4–5, 11; Africa and,
  3; consequences for society, 13;
  dangers of, 46; effects on family,
  11; incidence, 3–4; media and,
  14–17; medical complications
  of, 63; options for, 21–23;
  prevention and, 17; risk factors
  for, 4; self-esteem and, 5; social
  issue, 3–20
Temporary Assistance for Needy
  Families (TANF), 39
Third trimester, 49–50
Title IX, 39
Transition, 57. *See also* Labor
Truancy, 103; laws and, 103

Unemployment, 7
Unexpected, 15
Uterine ballottement, 45
Uterine contractions, 53–55. *See also*
  Labor

Vaccines for newborns, 66
Vacuum aspiration, 25–26; procedure
  for, 25; side effects, 25. *See also*
  Abortion
Violence, 7

Weatherization Assistance Program,
  41
Welfare, 8, 40, 42
Women, Infants, and Children
  (WIC), 38

About the Author

Paul Quinn, PhD, is a certified nurse midwife and women's health nurse practitioner and a national expert and speaker on issues surrounding women's health, obstetrics, and nursing workforce issues. His other works include Greenwood's *Sexually Transmitted Diseases: Your Questions Answered* and *Birth Control: Your Questions Answered.*